Repositioning Nutrition as Central to Development

A Strategy for Large-Scale Action

 THE WORLD BANK

Cover design by Fletcher Design
Cover photos by World Bank

ISBN-10: 0-8213-6399-9
ISBN-13: 978-0-8213-6399-7
eISBN-10: 0-8213-6400-6
eISBN-13: 978-0-8213-6400-0
DOI: 10.1596-978-0-8213-6399-7

For additional information, contact
Meera Shekar, HDNHE, World Bank

Contents

Tables

Figures

Boxes

Maps

"Nearly 4 million people die prematurely in India every year from malnutrition and related problems. That's more than the number who perished during the entire Bengal famine."

—Amartya Sen and Jean Dreze, Hunger and Public Action, 1989

"The portion of the global burden of disease (mortality and morbidity, 1990 figures) in developing countries that would be removed by eliminating malnutrition is estimated as 32 percent. This includes the effects of malnutrition on the most vulnerable groups' burden of mortality and morbidity from infectious diseases only. This is therefore a conservative figure..."

—John Mason, Philip Musgrove, and Jean-Pierre Habicht, 2003

"... investments in micronutrients have higher returns than those from investments in trade liberalization, in malaria, or in water and sanitation.... *No other technology offers as large an opportunity to improve lives at such low cost and in such a short time.*"

—Copenhagen Consensus, 2004

"Micronutrient deficiencies alone may cost India US$2.5 billion annually and the productivity losses (manual work only) from stunting, iodine deficiency, and iron deficiency together are responsible for a total loss of 2.95 percent of GDP."

—S. Horton, 1999

"Noncommunicable diseases account for almost 60 percent of the 56 million deaths annually and 47 percent of the global burden of disease...the burden of mortality, morbidity, and disability attributable to noncommunicable diseases is currently greatest and continuing to grow in the developing countries, where 66 percent of these deaths occur... the most important risks included high blood pressure, high concentrations of cholesterol in the blood, inadequate intake of fruits and vegetables, overweight or obesity, and physical inactivity that are closely related to diet and physical activity."

—WHO, 2004

"By 2002, only East Asia and Pacific and Latin America and the Caribbean had fewer undernourished people than 10 years earlier."

—World Bank, 2005a

"Sub-Saharan Africa is not on track to achieve a single MDG. ... it is off track on the hunger goal—and is the only region where child malnutrition is not declining.... And while malnutrition in the (South Asia) region is dropping sufficiently to achieve the MDG target reduction, *it remains at very high absolute levels:* almost half of children under five are underweight."

—World Bank, 2005b

"A hungry person is an angry and dangerous person. It is in all our interests to take away the cause of this anger."

—President Olusegun Obasanjo of Nigeria, *The Guardian*, June 23, 2005 (UK)

Foreword

Malnutrition remains the world's most serious health problem and the single biggest contributor to child mortality. Nearly one-third of children in the developing world are either underweight or stunted, and more than 30 percent of the developing world's population suffers from micronutrient deficiencies. Unless policies and priorities are changed, the scale of the problem will prevent many countries from achieving the Millennium Development Goals (MDGs)—especially in Sub-Saharan Africa, where malnutrition is increasing, and in South Asia, where malnutrition is widespread and improving only slowly.

There are also new dimensions to the malnutrition problem. The epidemic of obesity and diet-related noncommunicable diseases (NCDs) in developed countries is spreading to the developing world. Many poorer countries are now beginning to suffer from a double burden of undernutrition and obesity. This phenomenon, which some have termed the "nutrition transition," means that those national health systems now have to cope with the high cost of treating diet-related NCDs at the same time they are fighting undernutrition and the traditional, communicable diseases. Malnutrition is also linked to the growing HIV/AIDS pandemic; malnutrition makes adults more susceptible to the virus, inadequate infant feeding aggravates its transmission from mother to child; and evidence suggests that malnutrition makes antiretroviral drugs less effective.

Two developments, one negative and one positive, have led to this report at this juncture. The first is the growing international awareness that many MDGs will not be reached unless malnutrition is tackled, and that this continued failure of the development community to tackle malnutrition may derail other international efforts in health and in poverty reduction. The second development is the now unequivocal evidence that there are workable solutions to the malnutrition problem and that they are excellent economic investments. The May 2004 Copenhagen Consensus of eminent economists (including several Nobel laureates) concluded that the returns of investing in micronutrient programs are second only to the returns of fighting HIV/AIDS among a lengthy list of ways to meet the world's development challenges. Other nutrition-related interventions placed within the top dozen proposals.

There is also clear evidence that the major damage caused by malnutrition takes place in the womb and during the first two years of life; that this damage is irreversible; that it causes lower intelligence and reduced physical capacity, which in turn reduce productivity, slow economic growth, and perpetuate poverty; and that malnutrition passes from generation to generation because stunted mothers are more likely to have underweight children. This report sends the message that, to break this cycle, the focus must be on preventing and treating malnutrition among pregnant women and children aged zero to two years. School feeding programs—often sold as nutrition interventions—may help get children into school and keep them there, but such programs do not attack the malnutrition problem at its roots.

This report argues that there are long and short routes to improving nutrition. Higher incomes and better food security improve nutrition over the longer term, but malnutrition is not simply the result of food insecurity: many children in food-secure environments are underweight or stunted because of inappropriate infant feeding and care practices, poor access to health services, or poor sanitation. Much more attention therefore needs to be given to shorter routes to better nutrition—providing health and nutrition education and micronutrient fortification and supplementation. In addition, more attention needs to be directed to gender issues such as pregnant women's care of themselves and their children. Conditional cash transfers, when coupled with improvements in service quality and access, are a good way to get poor people to use nutrition services. This report provides a framework to help countries decide what nutrition actions are appropriate under different circumstances. It also presents epidemiological data in a user-friendly way to help development partners prioritize countries for support, though it emphasizes that country commitment and capacity—as well as need—should determine investment priorities.

Improving nutrition is not just about investing more. Equally important are conducting sound policy analysis, ensuring that nutrition policies are linked to nutrition action, and developing the appropriate capacity and institutional arrangements to manage nutrition programs. Strengthening commitment to tackling malnutrition and forging new partnerships to do so are critical to making progress—partnerships between governments, communities, and nongovernmental organizations; between governments and the development partner community; and between governments and the corporate sector, whose role in fortifying food and in taking responsibility for the nutritional content of snacks and fast food will be central.

Putting an end to extreme malnutrition will lay the foundation for improving the health and well-being of the present generation and lead to benefits for future generations over the 21st century. Nutrition is the true foundation of sustainable poverty reduction, yet it is still neglected. It is time to spread a broader awareness of the worldwide challenges of nutrition—and its links with health and sustainable development—and of the new opportunities for making global progress.

This report is written primarily for the community of international development partners, as well as those in government and civil society concerned with action to improve nutrition. It provides a global framework for action and complements similar analyses undertaken by the World Bank's regional units for Africa and South Asia. It is hoped that the report will reinvigorate dialogue regarding what to do about malnutrition; that it will encourage the development community to reevaluate the priority it gives nutrition; and that it will result in agreement on new ways for stakeholders to work together and in a new global commitment to scaling up proven interventions for tackling malnutrition.

As the Bank gears up to move nutrition higher on the development agenda, this report allows us to underline the importance of investing in nutrition.

Jacques Baudouy
Director, Health, Nutrition, and
   Population
Human Development Network

Jean-Louis Sarbib
Senior Vice President
Human Development Network

Acknowledgments

This document was produced by a team led by Meera Shekar, with Richard Heaver and Yi-Kyoung Lee. Milla McLachlan led the concept review process. Substantive inputs were provided by Judith McGuire and Savitha Subramanian. Kei Kawabata (sector manager of Health, Nutrition, and Population) provided valuable guidance and support throughout the development of the report.

The authors are grateful to Jean-Louis Sarbib, senior vice president of the World Bank's Human Development Network, and Jacques Baudouy, director of Health, Nutrition, and Population for their strategic support in repositioning the nutrition agenda in the World Bank.

Detailed peer review comments were provided on various versions of the report by Jere Behrman (University of Pennsylvania), Alan Berg, Venkatesh Mannar (Micronutrient Initiative), David Pelletier (Cornell University), Ellen Piwoz (Academy for Educational Development/Linkages), and Richard Skolnik (U.S. President's Emergency Fund for AIDS Relief), as well as Harold Alderman, Shanta Devarajan, John Fiedler, Paul Gertler, Michele Gragnolati, Keith Hansen, Kees Kostermans, Kathy Lindert, Claudia Rokx, Richard Seifman, and Susan Stout from the World Bank.

Several other colleagues attended review meetings and provided additional input and feedback during development of the report: Catherine Le Galès Camus (World Health Organization), Denise Coitinho (WHO), Frances Davidson (USAID), Stuart Gillespie (IFPRI), Marcia Griffiths (The Manoff Group), Rainer Gross (UNICEF), Jean-Pierre Habicht (Cornell University), Lawrence Haddad (Institute for Development Studies), Carol Marshall (Micronutrient Initiative), Roger Shrimpton (UN Standing Committee on Nutrition), and Lisa Studdert (Asian Development Bank), as well as Anabela Abreu, Jock Anderson, Lynn Brown, Barbara Bruns, Derek Byerlee, Mariam Claeson, Carlo Del Ninno, Jed Friedman, Rae Galloway, Charles Griffin, Pablo Gottret, Sabrina Huffman, Emmanuel Jimenez, Lucia Kossarova, Antonio Lim, Akiko Maeda, Tawhid Nawaz, Willyanne Del Cormier Plosby, Meera Priyadarshi, Julian Schweitzer,

Suneeta Singh, Kimberly Switlick, Chris Walker, and Evangeline Javier from the World Bank.

The report was edited by Bruce Ross-Larsen and his team at Communications Development, Inc.

Consultations with development partners provided guidance for the report. Additional consultations are planned in 2006.

The work was supported in part by a generous contribution from the Government of the Netherlands through the Bank-Netherlands Partnership Program grant to the World Bank.

Acronyms and Abbreviations

ADB	Asian Development Bank
AED	Academy for Educational Development
AFR	Africa Region
AIN-C	Atención Integral a la Niñez-Comunitaria
BASICS	Basic Support for Institutionalizing Child Survival
BINP	Bangladesh Integrated Nutrition Project
BMI	body mass index
BRAC	Bangladesh Rural Advancement Committee
CDD	community-driven development
CGIAR	Consultative Group on International Agricultural Research
CIDA	Canadian International Development Agency
DALY	disability-adjusted life years
DANIDA	Danish International Development Agency
DFID	U.K. Department for International Development
DGF	Development Grant Facility (World Bank)
DMC	developing member country
EAP	East Asia and the Pacific
EBF	exclusive breastfeeding
EC	European Commission
ECA	Eastern Europe and Central Asia
ECD	early childhood development
ENA	Essential Nutrition Actions
ESHE	Ethiopia Child Survival and Systems Strengthening Project
EU	European Union
FAD	Food Aid for Development
FANTA	Food and Nutrition Technical Assistance Project (USAID)
FAO	Food and Agricultural Organization (of the UN)
FFI	Fresh Food Initiative
GAIN	Global Alliance for Improving Nutrition
GDP	gross domestic product
GMP	Growth, Monitoring, and Promotion
GNI	gross national income

GNP	gross national product
GTZ	German Agency for Technical Assistance
HKI	Hellen Keller International
HNP	Health, Nutrition, and Population (World Bank)
HNPSP	Health, Nutrition, and Population Sector Program
HSD	Health systems development
ICDDR,B	International Centre for Diarrhoeal Disease Research, Bangladesh
ICDS	Integrated Child Development Services Program (India)
ICN	International Conference on Nutrition
IDA	iron deficiency anemia
IDD	iodine deficiency disorders
IEC	Information, Education, and Communication
IFAD	International Fund for Agricultural Development
IFPRI	International Food Policy Research Institute
IMCI	Integrated Management of Childhood Illnesses
JICA	Japanese International Co-operation Agency
KfW	German Development Bank
LAC	Latin America and the Caribbean
LDC	less developed country
MAP	Multicountry AIDS project
M&E	monitoring and evaluation
MDG	Millennium Development Goal
MENA	Middle East and North Africa
MI	Micronutrient Initiative
NCDs	noncommunicable diseases
NEPAD	New Partnership for Africa's Development
NESDB	National Economic and Social Development Board (Thailand)
NFA	National Food Authority
NGO	nongovernmental organizations
NHD	Nutrition for Health and Development
NID	National Immunization Day
OECD	Organisation for Economic Co-operation and Development
PEM	protein-energy malnutrition
PEPFAR	President's Emergency Plan for AIDS Relief
PRSCs	Poverty Reduction Strategy Credits
PRSPs	Poverty Reduction Strategy Papers
PSIA	Poverty and Social Impact Analysis
RENEWAL	Regional Network on HIV/AIDS, Rural Livelihoods, and Food Security
SAR	South Asia Region
SARA	Support for Analysis and Research in Africa

SCN   Standing Committee on Nutrition
SIDA   Swedish International Development Agency
SWAP   sectorwide approach
TINP   Tamil Nadu Integrated Nutrition Project
TIPs   trials of improved practices (USAID)
UNFPA   United Nations Fund for Population Activities
UNICEF   United Nations Children's Fund
USAID   United States Agency for International Development
VAD   vitamin A deficiency
WABA   World Alliance for Breastfeeding Action
WFP   World Food Program
WFS   World Food Summit
WHO   World Health Organization

All dollar amounts are U.S. dollars unless otherwise indicated.

Glossary

Anemia	Low level of hemoglobin in the blood, as evidenced by a reduced quality or quantity of red blood cells; 50 percent of anemia worldwide is caused by iron deficiency.
Body mass index (BMI)	Body weight in kilograms divided by height in meters squared (kg/m^2). This is used as an index of "fatness." Both high BMI (overweight, BMI greater than 25) and low BMI (thinness, BMI less than 18.5) are considered inadequate.
Iodine deficiency disorders (IDDs)	All of the ill effects of iodine deficiency in a population that can be prevented by ensuring that the population has an adequate intake of iodine. The spectrum of IDD includes goiter, hypothyroidism, impaired mental function, stillbirths, abortions, congenital anomalies, and neurological cretinism.
Low birthweight	Birthweight less than 2,500 grams.
Malnutrition	Various forms of poor nutrition caused by a complex array of factors including dietary inadequacy, infections, and sociocultural factors. Underweight or stunting and overweight, as well as micronutrient deficiencies, are forms of malnutrition.
Obesity	Excessive body fat content; commonly measured by BMI. The international reference for classifying an individual as obese is a BMI greater than 30.

Overweight

Excess weight relative to height; commonly measured by BMI among adults (see above). The international reference for adults is as follows:
- 25–29.99 for grade I (overweight).
- 30–39.99 for grade II (obese).
- > 40 for grade III.

For children, overweight is measured as weight-for-height two z-scores above the international reference.

Stunting (measured as height-for-age)

Failure to reach linear growth potential because of inadequate nutrition or poor health. It implies long-term undernutrition and poor health, measured as height-for-age two z-scores below the international reference. Usually a good indicator of long-term undernutrition among young children. For children under 12 months, recumbent length is used instead of height.

Undernutrition

Poor nutrition: It may occur in association with infection. Three most commonly used indexes for child undernutrition are height-for-age, weight-for-age, and weight-for-height. For adults, undernutrition is measured by a BMI less than 18.5.

Underweight

Low weight-for-age; that is, two z-scores below the international reference for weight-for-age. It implies stunting or wasting and is an indicator of undernutrition.

Vitamin A deficiency

Tissue concentrations of vitamin A low enough to have adverse health consequences such as increased morbidity and mortality, poor reproductive health, and slowed growth and development, even if there is no clinical deficiency.

Wasting (measured by weight-for-height)	Weight (in kilograms) divided by height (in meters squared) that is two z-scores below the international reference. It describes a recent or current severe process leading to significant weight loss, usually a consequence of acute starvation or severe disease. Commonly used as an indicator of undernutrition among children; especially useful in emergency situations such as famine.
z-score	The deviation of an individual's value from the median value of a reference population, divided by the standard deviation of the reference population.

Overview

It has long been known that malnutrition undermines economic growth and perpetuates poverty. Yet the international community and most governments in developing countries have failed to tackle malnutrition over the past decades, even though well-tested approaches for doing so exist. The consequences of this failure to act are now evident in the world's inadequate progress toward the Millennium Development Goals (MDGs) and toward poverty reduction more generally. Persistent malnutrition is contributing not only to widespread failure to meet the first MDG—to halve poverty and hunger—but to meet other goals in maternal and child health, HIV/AIDS, education, and gender equity. The unequivocal choice now is between continuing to fail, as the global community did with HIV/AIDS for more than a decade, or to finally make nutrition central to development so that a wide range of economic and social improvements that depend on nutrition can be realized.

Three Reasons for Intervening to Reduce Malnutrition

High economic returns; high impact on economic growth and poverty reduction

The returns to investing in nutrition are very high. The Copenhagen Consensus concluded that nutrition interventions generate returns among the highest of 17 potential development investments (table 1). Investments in micronutrients were rated above those in trade liberalization, malaria, and water and sanitation. Community-based programs targeted to children under two years of age are also cost-effective in preventing undernutrition.

Overall, the benefit-cost ratios for nutrition interventions range between 5 and 200 (table 2).

Malnutrition slows economic growth and perpetuates poverty through three routes—direct losses in productivity from poor physical status; indirect losses from poor cognitive function and deficits in schooling; and losses

Table 1 The Copenhagen Consensus ranks the provision of micronutrients as a top investment

Rating	Challenge	Opportunity
Very good	1. Diseases	Controlling HIV/AIDS
	2. Malnutrition and hunger	Providing micronutrients
	3. Subsidies and trade	Liberalizing trade
	4. Diseases	Controlling malaria
Good	5. Malnutrition and hunger	Developing new agricultural technologies
	6. Sanitation and water	Developing small-scale water technologies
	7. Sanitation and water	Implementing community-managed systems
	8. Sanitation and water	Conducting research on water in agriculture
	9. Government	Lowering costs of new business
Fair	10. Migration	Lowering barriers to migration
	11. Malnutrition and hunger	Improving infant and child malnutrition
	12. Diseases	Scaling up basic health services
	13. Malnutrition and hunger	Reducing the prevalence of low birthweight
Poor	14–17. Climate/migration	Various

Source: Bhagwati and others (2004).

owing to increased health care costs. Malnutrition's economic costs are substantial: productivity losses to individuals are estimated at more than 10 percent of lifetime earnings, and gross domestic product (GDP) lost to malnutrition runs as high as 2 to 3 percent. Improving nutrition is therefore as much—or more—of an issue of economics as one of welfare, social protection, and human rights.

Reducing undernutrition and micronutrient malnutrition directly reduces poverty, in the broad definition that includes human development and human capital formation. But undernutrition is also strongly linked to income poverty. The prevalence of malnutrition is often two or three times—sometimes many times—higher among the poorest income quintile than among the highest quintile. This means that improving nutrition is a pro-poor strategy, disproportionately increasing the income-earning potential of the poor.

Table 2 The benefit-cost ratios for nutrition programs

Intervention programs	Benefit-cost
Breastfeeding promotion in hospitals	5–67
Integrated child care programs	9–16
Iodine supplementation (women)	15–520
Vitamin A supplementation (children < 6 years)	4–43
Iron fortification (per capita)	176–200
Iron supplementation (per pregnant women)	6–14

Source: Behrman, Alderman, and Hoddinott (2004).

Improving nutrition is essential to reduce extreme poverty. Recognition of this requirement is evident in the definition of the first MDG, which aims to eradicate extreme poverty and hunger. The two targets are to halve, between 1990 and 2015:

- The proportion of people whose income is less than $1 a day.
- The proportion of people who suffer from hunger (as measured by the percentage of children under five who are underweight).

The first target refers to income poverty; the second addresses nonincome poverty. The key indicator used for measuring progress on the nonincome poverty goal is the prevalence of underweight children (under age five).Therefore, improving nutrition is in itself an MDG target. Yet most assessments of progress toward the MDGs have focused primarily on the income poverty target, and the prognosis in general is that most countries are on track for achieving the poverty goal. But of 143 countries, only 34 (24 percent) are on track to achieve the nonincome target (nutrition MDG) (figure 1). No country in South Asia, where undernutrition is the highest, will achieve the MDG—though Bangladesh will come close to achieving it, and Asia as a whole will achieve it. More alarmingly still, nutrition status is actually deteriorating in 26 countries, many of them in Africa, where the nexus between HIV and undernutrition is particularly strong and mutually reinforcing. And in 57 countries, no trend data are available to tell whether progress is being made. A renewed focus on this nonincome poverty target is clearly central to any poverty reduction efforts.

The alarming shape and scale of the malnutrition problem

Malnutrition is now a problem in both poor and rich countries, with the poorest people in both sets of countries affected most. In developed countries, obesity is rapidly becoming more widespread, especially among

Figure 1 Progress toward the nonincome poverty target

On track (24%)		Deteriorating status (18%)	
AFR (7)	**LAC (10)**	**AFR (13)**	**ECA (4)**
Angola	Bolivia	Niger	Albania
Benin	Chile	Burkina Faso	Azerbaijan
Botswana	Colombia	Cameroon	Russian Federation
Chad	Dominican Rep.	Comoros	Serbia and Montenegro
Gambia, The	Guyana	Ethiopia	
Mauritania	Haiti	Guinea	**LAC (3)**
Zimbabwe	Jamaica	Lesotho	Argentina
	Mexico	Mali	Costa Rica
EAP (5)	Peru	Senegal*	Panama
China	Venezuela, R.B. de	Sudan	
Indonesia		Tanzania*	**MENA (2)**
Malaysia	**MENA (6)**	Togo	Iraq
Thailand	Algeria	Zambia	Yemen, Rep. of
Vietnam	Egypt, Arab Rep. of		
	Iran, Islamic	**EAP (2)**	**SAR (2)**
ECA (6)	Rep. of Jordan	Mongolia	Maldives
Armenia	Syrian Arab Rep.	Myanmar	Nepal
Croatia	Tunisia		
Kazakhstan			
Kyrgyz Rep.	**SAR (0)**		
Romania		**No trend data available (40%)**	
Turkey			
		AFR (13)	Georgia
		Burundi	Hungary
		Cape Verde	Latvia
Some improvement, but not on track		Congo, Rep. of	Lithuania
		Equatorial Guinea	Macedonia, FYR
AFR (14)		Guinea	Moldova
Central African Rep.	**ECA (0)**	Guinea-Bissau	Poland
Congo, DR		Liberia	Slovak Republic
Côte d'Ivoire	**LAC (4)**	Mauritius	Tajikistan
Eritrea	El Salvador	Namibia	Turkmenistan
Gabon	Guatemala	Sâo Tomé and Principe	Ukraine
Ghana	Honduras	Seychelles	Uzbekistan
Kenya	Nicaragua	Somalia	
Madagascar		South Africa	**LAC (12)**
Malawi	**MENA (1)**	Swaziland	Belize
Mozambique	Morocco		Brazil
Nigeria		**EAP (11)**	Dominica
Rwanda	**SAR (4)**	Fiji	Ecuador
Sierra Leone	Bangladesh*	Kiribati	Grenada
Uganda	India	Marshall Is.	Paraguay
	Pakistan	Micronesia, Federated	St. Kitts and Nevis
EAP (5)	Sri Lanka	States of	St. Lucia
Cambodia		Palau	St. Vincent
Lao PDR		Papua New Guinea	Suriname
Phillippines		Samoa	Trinidad and Tobago
		Solomon Islands	Uruguay
		Timor-Leste	
		Tonga	**MENA (2)**
		Vanuatu	Djibouti
			Lebanon
		ECA (17)	
		Belarus	**SAR (2)**
		Bosnia and	Afghanistan
		Herzegovina	Bhutan
		Bulgaria	
		Czech Republic	
		Estonia	

Source: Author's calculations. See also technical annex 5.6.

Note: All calculations are based on 1990–2002 trend data from the WHO Global Database on Child Growth and Malnutrition (as of April 2005). Countries indicated by an asterisk subsequently released preliminary DHS data that suggest improvement and therefore may be reclassified when their data are officially released.

Figure 2 Prevalence of and trends in malnutrition among children under age five, 1980–2005

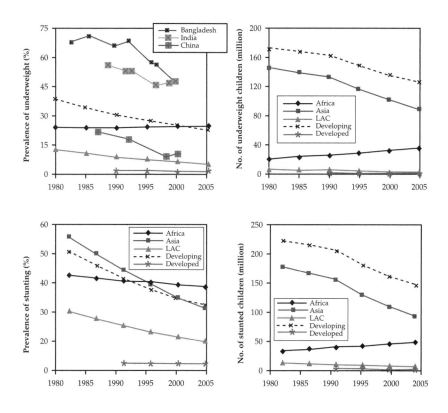

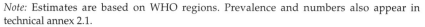

Source: De Onis (2004a); SCN (2004).
Note: Estimates are based on WHO regions. Prevalence and numbers also appear in technical annex 2.1.

poorer people, bringing with it an epidemic of diet-related noncommunicable diseases (NCDs) such as diabetes and heart disease, which increase health care costs and reduce productivity. In developing countries, while widespread undernutrition and micronutrient deficiencies persist, obesity is also fast emerging as a problem. Underweight children and overweight adults are now often found in the same households in both developing and developed countries.

Nearly one-third of children in the developing world remain underweight or stunted, and 30 percent of the developing world's population

Figure 3 Projected trends in numbers of underweight children under age five, 1990–2015

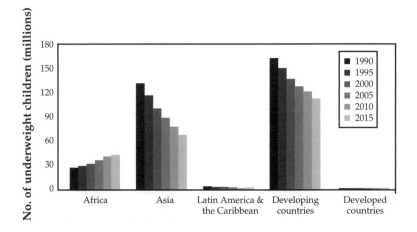

Source: De Onis and others (2004a, 2004b).
Note: Estimates are based on WHO regions.

continues to suffer from micronutrient deficiencies. But the picture is chang-ing (figure 2):

- In Sub-Saharan Africa malnutrition is on the rise. Malnutrition and HIV/AIDS reinforce each other, so the success of HIV/AIDS programs in Africa depends in part on paying more attention to nutrition.
- In Asia malnutrition is decreasing, but South Asia still has both the high-est rates and the largest numbers of malnourished children. Contrary to common perceptions, undernutrition prevalence rates in the popu-lous South Asian countries—India, Bangladesh, Afghanistan, Pakistan—are much higher (38 to 51 percent) than those in Sub-Saharan Africa (26 percent).
- Even in East Asia, Latin America, and Eastern Europe, many countries have a serious problem of undernutrition or micronutrient malnutri-tion. Examples include Cambodia, Indonesia, Lao PDR, the Philippines, and Vietnam; Guatemala, Haiti, and Honduras; and Uzbekistan.

In a recent WHO study (De Onis and others 2004b), underweight preva-lence in developing countries was forecast to decline by 36 percent (from 30 percent in 1990 to 19 percent in 2015)—significantly below the 50 per-cent required to meet the MDG over the same time frame (figure 3).[1] These global data mask interregional differences that are widening disturbingly. Much of the forecast global improvement derives from a projected prevalence decline from 35 to 18 percent in Asia—driven primarily by the improvements in China. By contrast, in Africa, the prevalence is projected to increase from 24 to 27 percent. And the situation in Eastern Africa—a region blighted by HIV/AIDS, which has major interactions with malnutrition—is critical. Here underweight prevalences are forecast to be 25 percent higher in 2015 than they were in 1990.

Many countries (excluding several in Sub-Saharan Africa) will achieve the MDG income poverty target (percentage of people living on less than $1 a day), but less than 25 percent will achieve the nonincome poverty target of halving underweight (figure 3). Even if Asia as a whole achieves that target, large countries there including Afghanistan, Bangladesh, India, and Pakistan will still have unacceptably high rates of undernutrition in 2015, widening existing inequities between the rich and the poor in these countries.

Deficiencies of key vitamins and minerals continue to be pervasive, and they overlap considerably with problems of general undernutrition (underweight and stunting). A recent global progress report states that 35 percent of people in the world lack adequate iodine, 40 percent of people in the developing world suffer from iron deficiency, and more than 40 percent of children are vitamin A deficient.

Trends in overweight among children under five, though based on data from a limited number of countries, are alarming (figure 4)—for all developing countries and particularly for those in Africa, where rates seem to be increasing at a far greater rate (58 percent increase) than in the developing world as a whole (17 percent increase). The lack of data does not allow us to give definitive answers for why Africa is experiencing this exaggerated trend; however, the correlation between maternal overweight and child overweight suggests that one of the answers may lie therein.

Comparable data for overweight and obesity rates among mothers show similar alarming trends. Countries in the Middle East and North Africa have the highest maternal overweight rates, followed by those in Latin America and the Caribbean. However, several African countries have more than 20 percent maternal overweight rates.

Also evident is that overweight coexists in the same countries where both child and maternal undernutrition are very widespread and in many countries with low per capita GNP (figure 5). In Mauritania, more than 40 percent of mothers are overweight, while at the same time more than 30 percent children are underweight. Furthermore, as many as 60 percent of households with an underweight person also had an overweight person, demonstrating that underweight and overweight coexist not only in the same countries but also in the same households. In Guatemala, stunted children and over-

weight mothers coexist. Again, these data support the premise that, except
under famine conditions, access to and availability of food at the household level are not the major causes of undernutrition.

Figure 4 Trends in obesity among children under age five

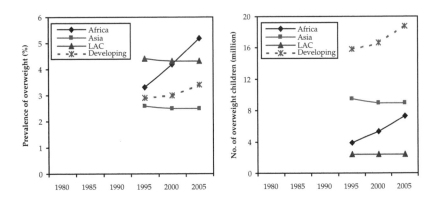

Source: SCN (2004).
Note: Estimates are based on WHO regions.

Figure 5 Maternal overweight rates across regions

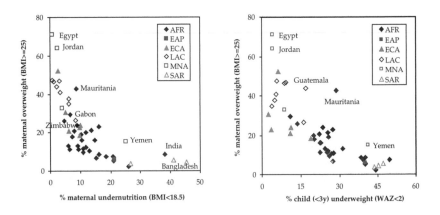

Source: Author's calculations using data from measuredhs.com.

Markets are failing

Markets are failing to address the malnutrition problem wherever families do not have the money to buy adequate food or health care. Human rights and equity arguments, as well as economic return arguments, can be made for governments to intervene to help such families. But malnutrition occurs also in many families that are not poor—because people do not always know what food or feeding practices are best for their children or themselves, and because people cannot easily tell when their children are becoming malnourished, since faltering growth rates and micronutrient deficiencies are not usually visible to the untrained eye. The need to correct these "informational asymmetries" is another argument for government intervention (box 1). And governments should intervene because improved nutrition is a public good, benefiting everybody; for example, better nutrition can reduce the spread of contagious diseases and increase national economic productivity.

Box 1 Why malnutrition persists in many food-secure households

- Pregnant and nursing women eat too few calories and too little protein, have untreated infections, such as sexually transmitted diseases that lead to low birthweight, or do not get enough rest.
- Mothers have too little time to take care of their young children or themselves during pregnancy.
- Mothers of newborns discard colostrum, the first milk, which strengthens the child's immune system.
- Mothers often feed children under age 6 months foods other than breast milk even though exclusive breastfeeding is the best source of nutrients and the best protection against many infectious and chronic diseases.
- Caregivers start introducing complementary solid foods too late.
- Caregivers feed children under age two years too little food, or foods that are not energy dense.
- Though food is available, because of inappropriate household food allocation, women and young children's needs are not met and their diets often do not contain enough of the right micronutrients or protein.
- Caregivers do not know how to feed children during and following diarrhea or fever.
- Caregivers' poor hygiene contaminates food with bacteria or parasites.

What Causes Malnutrition and
How Should Governments Intervene?

Contrary to popular perceptions, undernutrition is not simply a result of food insecurity: many children in food-secure environments and from non-poor families are underweight or stunted because of inappropriate infant feeding and care practices, poor access to health services, or poor sanitation. In many countries where malnutrition is widespread, food production is not the limiting factor (box 2), except under famine conditions. The most important factors are, first, inadequate knowledge about the benefits of exclusive breastfeeding and complementary feeding practices and the role of micronutrients and second, the lack of time women have available for appropriate infant care practices and their own care during pregnancy.

Undernutrition's most damaging effect occurs during pregnancy and in the first two years of life, and the effects of this early damage on health, brain development, intelligence, educability, and productivity are largely irreversible (box 3). Actions targeted to older children have little, if any effect. Initial evidence suggests that the origins of obesity and NCDs such as cardiovascular heart disease and diabetes may also lie in early childhood. Governments with limited resources are therefore best advised to focus actions on this small window of opportunity, between conception and 24 months of age, although actions to control obesity may need to continue later.

In countries where mean overweight rates among children under age five are high, a large proportion of children are already overweight at birth—suggesting again that the damage happens in pregnancy. These results are consistent with physiological evidence that the origins of obesity start very early in life, often in the womb, though interventions to prevent obesity must likely continue in later life.

Income growth and food production, as well as birth spacing and women's education, are therefore important but long routes to improving nutrition. Shorter routes are providing health and nutrition education and services (such as promoting exclusive breastfeeding and appropriate complementary feeding, coupled with prenatal care and basic maternal and child health services) and micronutrient supplementation and fortification. Experience in Mexico shows that in middle-income countries conditional cash transfers, coupled with improved health and nutrition service delivery on the supply side, have gotten poor people to use nutrition services. Other countries, such as Bangladesh, Honduras, and Madagascar, have successfully used government-nongovernment partnerships to mobilize communities to tackle malnutrition through community-based approaches.

Experience in dealing with different forms of malnutrition is at different stages of development:

Box 2 Three myths about nutrition

Poor nutrition is implicated in more than half of all child deaths world-wide—a proportion unmatched by any infectious disease since the Black Death. It is intimately linked with poor health and environmental factors. But planners, politicians, and economists often fail to recognize these connections. Serious misapprehensions include the following myths:

Myth 1: *Malnutrition is primarily a matter of inadequate food intake.* Not so. Food is of course important. But most serious malnutrition is caused by bad sanitation and disease, leading to diarrhea, especially among young children. Women's status and women's education play big parts in improving nutrition. Improving care of young children is vital.

Myth 2: *Improved nutrition is a by-product of other measures of poverty reduction and economic advance. It is not possible to jump-start the process.* Again, untrue. Improving nutrition requires focused action by parents and communities, backed by local and national action in health and public services, especially water and sanitation. Thailand has shown that moderate and severe malnutrition can be reduced by 75 percent or more in a decade by such means.

Myth 3: *Given scarce resources, broad-based action on nutrition is hardly feasible on a mass scale, especially in poor countries.* Wrong again. In spite of severe economic setbacks, many developing countries have made impressive progress. More than two-thirds of the people in developing countries now eat iodized salt, combating the iodine deficiency and anemia that affect about 3.5 billion people, especially women and children in some 100 nations. About 450 million children a year now receive vitamin A capsules, tackling the deficiency that causes blindness and increases child mortality. New ways have been found to promote and support breastfeeding, and breastfeeding rates are being maintained in many countries and increased in some. Mass immunization and promotion of oral rehydration to reduce deaths from diarrhea have also done much to improve nutrition.

Source: Extracted from Jolly (1996).

- For undernutrition and micronutrient malnutrition, several large-scale programs have worked (in Bangladesh and Thailand, in Madagascar, and in Chile, Cuba, Honduras, and Mexico). The challenge is to apply their lessons at scale in more countries. The issue is less about what to do than about how to strengthen both countries' and development partners' commitment and capacity to scale up.

Box 3 The window of opportunity for addressing undernutrition

The window of opportunity for improving nutrition is small—from before pregnancy through the first two years of life. There is consensus that the damage to physical growth, brain development, and human capital formation that occurs during this period is extensive and largely irreversible. Therefore interventions must focus on this window of opportunity. Any investments after this critical period are much less likely to improve nutrition.

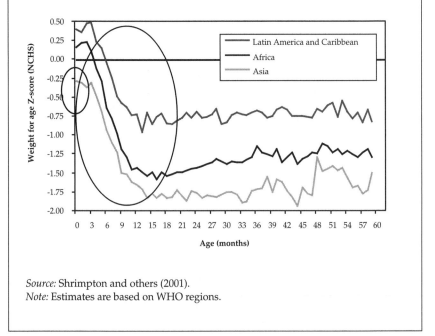

Source: Shrimpton and others (2001).
Note: Estimates are based on WHO regions.

- By contrast, for overweight and diet-related NCDs, low birthweight, and the complex interactions between malnutrition and HIV/AIDS, there are few tried and tested large-scale models. Action research and learning-by-doing are the priority here, but large-scale HIV or NCD control efforts cannot be successful without addressing nutrition—so the challenge is to shorten the time lag between developing the science and scaling up action.

Although some successful programs have been scaled up without comprehensive nutrition policies, policy is important as well. Few countries have well-developed and well-resourced nutrition policies. More often, policies in other sectors (trade, foreign exchange, employment, gender, agriculture, social welfare, and health) have a haphazard, sometimes negative effect on nutrition and become unintentional but de facto nutrition policies. Poverty and Social Impact Analyses (PSIAs) should be more widely used to assess the intentional and unintentional effects of development policies on nutrition outcomes. And the capacity to advise policy makers about the nutrition implications of policy needs to be developed in a focal institution, such as a ministry of finance or a poverty monitoring office.

Policy also has a potential role in diminishing the poor health and negative economic outcomes associated with the increase in overweight and obesity in developing countries through both demand-side and supply-side interventions.

If effective interventions exist, why have they not been scaled up in more countries?

Nutrition programs have been low priority for both governments and development partners for three reasons (box 5). First, there is little demand for nutrition services from communities because malnutrition is often invisible; families and communities are unaware that even moderate and mild malnutrition contributes substantially to death, disease, and low intelligence; and most malnourished families are poor and hence have little voice. Second, governments and development partners have been slow to recognize how high malnutrition's economic costs are, that malnutrition is holding back progress not only toward the malnutrition MDG but also toward other MDGs, or that there is now substantial experience with how to implement cost-effective, affordable nutrition programs on a large scale. Third, there are multiple organizational stakeholders in nutrition, so malnutrition often falls between the cracks both in governments and in development assistance agencies—the partial responsibility of several sectoral ministries or agency departments, but the main responsibility of none. Country financing is usually allocated by sectors or ministries, so unless one sector takes the lead, no large-scale action can follow.

How the international development community can help countries do more

Countries need to take the lead in repositioning nutrition much higher in their development agenda. When countries request help in nutrition, development partners must respond first by helping countries develop a shared

---

**Box 5 Ten reasons for weak commitment
to nutrition programs**

- Malnutrition is usually invisible to malnourished families and communities.
- Families and governments do not recognize the human and economic costs of malnutrition.
- Governments may not know there are faster interventions for combating malnutrition than economic growth and poverty reduction or that nutrition programs are affordable.
- Because there are multiple organizational stakeholders in nutrition, it can fall between the cracks.
- There is not always a consensus about how to intervene against malnutrition.
- Adequate nutrition is seldom treated as a human right.
- The malnourished have little voice.
- Some politicians and managers do not care whether programs are well implemented.
- Governments sometimes claim they are investing in improving nutrition when the programs they are financing have little effect on it (for example, school feeding).
- A vicious circle: lack of commitment to nutrition leads to underinvestment in nutrition, which leads to weak impact, which reinforces lack of commitment since governments believe nutrition programs do not work.

Source: Abridged from Heaver (2005b).

---

vision and consensus on what needs to be done, how, and by whom, and then by providing financial and other assistance. This report argues that much of the failure to scale up action in nutrition results from a lack of sustained government commitment, leading to low demand for assistance in nutrition. In this situation, the role of development partners must extend beyond responding when requested to do so by governments. They must use their combined resources of analysis, advocacy, and capacity-building to encourage and influence governments to move nutrition higher on the agenda wherever it is holding back achievement of the MDGs (table 3). This role can be fulfilled only if the development partners share a common view of the malnutrition problem and broad strategies to address it, and if they speak with a common voice. The development partners therefore also need to reposition themselves. They need to convene around a common

Table 3 How investing in nutrition is critical to achieving the MDGs

Goal	Nutrition effect
Goal 1: Eradicate extreme poverty and hunger.	Malnutrition erodes human capital through irreversible and intergenerational effects on cognitive and physical development.
Goal 2: Achieve universal primary education.	Malnutrition affects the chances that a child will go to school, stay in school, and perform well.
Goal 3: Promote gender equality and empower women.	Antifemale biases in access to food, health, and care resources may result in malnutrition, possibly reducing women's access to assets. Addressing malnutrition empowers women more than men.
Goal 4: Reduce child mortality.	Malnutrition is directly or indirectly associated with most child deaths, and it is the main contributor to the burden of disease in the developing world.
Goal 5: Improve maternal health.	Maternal health is compromised by malnutrition, which is associated with most major risk factors for maternal mortality. Maternal stunting and iron and iodine deficiencies particularly pose serious problems.
Goal 6: Combat HIV/AIDS, malaria, and other diseases.	Malnutrition may increase risk of HIV transmission, compromise antiretroviral therapy, and hasten the onset of full-blown AIDS and premature death. It increases the chances of tuberculosis infection, resulting in disease, and it also reduces malarial survival rates.

Source: Adapted from Gillespie and Haddad (2003).

strategic agenda in nutrition, focusing on scaled-up and more effective action for undernutrition and micronutrients in priority countries and on action research or learning-by-doing for overweight, low birthweight, and HIV/AIDS and nutrition. This repositioning must involve reviewing and revising the current inadequate levels of funding for nutrition. For example, though the World Bank is the largest development partner investing in global nutrition, between 2000 and 2004 its investments in the short route interventions that improve nutrition fastest amounted to not more than 3.8 percent of its lending for human development—and less than 0.7 percent of total World Bank lending.

Although we do not wish to propose a global "one size fits all" approach to addressing malnutrition, we do recommend that when developing strategies specific to a country or region, countries and their development partners pay special attention to the following:

- Focusing strategies and actions on the poor so as to address the nonincome aspects of poverty reduction that are closely linked to human development and human capital formation.
- Focusing interventions on the window of opportunity—before pregnancy through the first two years of life—because this is when irreparable damage happens.
- Improving maternal and child care practices to reduce the incidence of low birthweight and to improve infant-feeding practices, including exclusive breastfeeding and appropriate and timely complementary feeding, because many countries and development partners have neglected to invest in such programs.
- Scaling up micronutrient programs because of their widespread prevalence, their effect on productivity, their affordability, and their extraordinarily high benefit-cost ratios.
- Building on country capacities developed through micronutrient programming to extend actions to community-based nutrition programs.
- Working to improve nutrition not only through health but also through appropriate actions in agriculture, rural development, water supply and sanitation, social protection, education, gender, and community-driven development.
- Strengthening investments in the short routes to improving nutrition, yet maintaining balance between the short and the long routes.
- Integrating appropriately designed and balanced nutrition actions in country assistance strategies, sectorwide approaches (SWAps) in multiple sectors, multicountry AIDS projects (MAPs), and Poverty Reduction Strategy Papers (PRSPs).

In addition to these generic recommendations, practical suggestions are available for how countries might take some of these considerations into account as they position nutrition in their national development strategies.

Next Steps

Scaled-up and more effective action requires addressing key operational challenges:

1. Building global and national commitment and capacity to invest in nutrition.
2. Mainstreaming nutrition in country development strategies where it is not now given priority.
3. Reorienting ineffective, large-scale nutrition programs to maximize their effect.

Action research and learning-by-doing need to focus on:

1. Documenting how best to strengthen commitment and capacity and to mainstream nutrition in the development agenda.
2. Strengthening and fine-tuning service delivery mechanisms for nutrition.
3. Further strengthening the evidence base for investing in nutrition.

At the global level, the development community needs to unite in explicitly rethinking and repositioning the role of malnutrition as an underlying cause of slow economic growth, mortality, and morbidity, and agree to:

- Coordinate efforts to strengthen commitment and funding for nutrition within global and national partnerships.
- Pursue a set of broad strategic priorities (such as the six outlined above) for the next decade, contributing wherever they have the most comparative advantage.
- Focus on an agreed-on set of priority countries for investing in nutrition and for mainstreaming and scaling up nutrition programs.
- Focus on an agreed-on set of priority countries for developing best practices in building commitment and capacity, mainstreaming nutrition, and reducing overweight and obesity.
- Make a collective effort to switch from financing small-scale projects to financing large-scale programs, except where small projects with strong monitoring and evaluation components are required to pilot-test interventions and delivery systems, or to build capacity in nutrition.

At the country level, the development community needs to scale up its assistance by helping all countries that have micronutrient deficiencies develop a national strategy for micronutrients, finance it, and scale it up to nationwide coverage within five years—without crowding out the larger undernutrition agenda.

The development community must also support countries with undernutrition problems as follows:

- Identify and support at least 5 to 10 countries with serious nutrition problems that have the commitment to work with development partners to mainstream nutrition into SWAps, MAPs, and Poverty Reduction Strategy Credits (PRSCs). In countries that have little experience in nutrition, nutrition projects may be the first step; in other cases, specific efforts to develop country capacity will be needed.
- Identify and support three to five countries where large-scale investments need to be reoriented to maximize their effect. In these countries, provide coordinated support to reorient program design and to strengthen implementation quality and monitoring and evaluation.
- Identify and support at least three to five countries where nutrition issues loom large but appropriate action is not being taken. In these countries, focus on building commitment, analyzing policy, and developing intervention strategies that can be financed with assistance from development partners.

To help achieve these goals, the development partners will need to cofinance a grant fund to catalyze action in commitment-building and action research, complementing the Bank's recent allocation of $3.6 million from the Development Grant Facility to help mainstream nutrition into maternal and child health programs. Large-scale funding for the national actions outlined above should come through normal financing channels, rather than through the creation of a special fund for nutrition. Initial estimates suggest that the costs of addressing the micronutrient agenda in Africa are approximately $235 million per year. Costs for other regions and for other aspects of the nutrition agenda have yet to be estimated. Other estimates are much larger ($750 million for global costs for two doses of Vitamin A supplementation per year; between $1 billion and $1.5 billion for global salt iodization, including $800 million to $1.2 billion leveraged from the private sector; and several billion dollars for community nutrition programs). A more detailed costing exercise is being undertaken by the World Bank to come up with more rigorous figures.

The agenda proposed here needs to be debated, modified, agreed on, and acted on by development partners with developing countries. Without coordinated, focused, and increased action, no significant progress in nutrition or toward several other MDGs can be expected.

Notes

1. De Onis and others (2004b).
2. Doak and others (2005).

Map 1.1 Global prevalence of underweight among children under age five

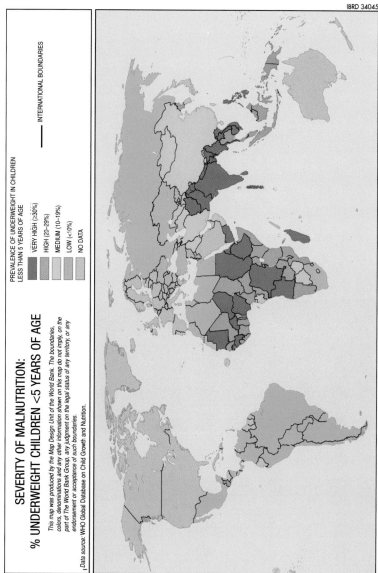

IBRD 34045

SEVERITY OF MALNUTRITION:
% UNDERWEIGHT CHILDREN <5 YEARS OF AGE

This map was produced by the Map Design Unit of the World Bank. The boundaries, colors, denominations and any other information shown on this map do not imply, on the part of The World Bank Group, any judgment on the legal status of any territory, or any endorsement or acceptance of such boundaries.

Data source: WHO Global Database on Child Growth and Nutrition.

PREVALENCE OF UNDERWEIGHT IN CHILDREN
LESS THAN 5 YEARS OF AGE

- VERY HIGH (≥30%)
- HIGH (20–29%)
- MEDIUM (10–19%)
- LOW (<10%)
- NO DATA

—— INTERNATIONAL BOUNDARIES

JULY 2005

Map 1.2 Prevalence of stunting in children less than five years of age

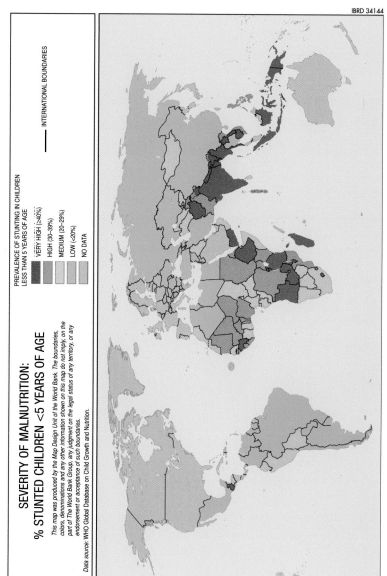

SEVERITY OF MALNUTRITION:
% STUNTED CHILDREN <5 YEARS OF AGE

This map was produced by the Map Design Unit of the World Bank. The boundaries,
colors, denominations and any other information shown on this map do not imply, on the
part of The World Bank Group, any judgment on the legal status of any territory, or any
endorsement or acceptance of such boundaries.

Data source: WHO Global Database on Child Growth and Nutrition.

PREVALENCE OF STUNTING IN CHILDREN
LESS THAN 5 YEARS OF AGE

- VERY HIGH (≥40%)
- HIGH (30–39%)
- MEDIUM (20–29%)
- LOW (<20%)
- NO DATA

—— INTERNATIONAL BOUNDARIES

IBRD 34144

JULY 2005

Map 1.3 Global prevalence of vitamin A deficiency and supplementation coverage rates

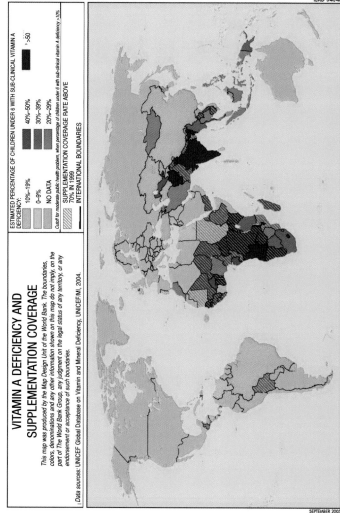

VITAMIN A DEFICIENCY AND SUPPLEMENTATION COVERAGE

This map was produced by the Map Design Unit of the World Bank. The boundaries, colors, denominations and any other information shown on this map do not imply, on the part of The World Bank Group, any judgment on the legal status of any territory, or any endorsement or acceptance of such boundaries.

Data sources: UNICEF Global Database on Vitamin and Mineral Deficiency, UNICEF/MI, 2004.

ESTIMATED PERCENTAGE OF CHILDREN UNDER 6 WITH SUB-CLINICAL VITAMIN A DEFICIENCY:

- 10%–19%
- 0–9%
- NO DATA
- 40%–50%
- 30%–39%
- 20%–29%
- >50

Cutoff for moderate public health problem, when percentage of children under 6 with sub-clinical vitamin A deficiency >10%

SUPPLEMENTATION COVERAGE RATE ABOVE 70% IN 1999

INTERNATIONAL BOUNDARIES

Map 1.4 Global prevalence of iodine deficiency disorders and iodized salt coverage rates

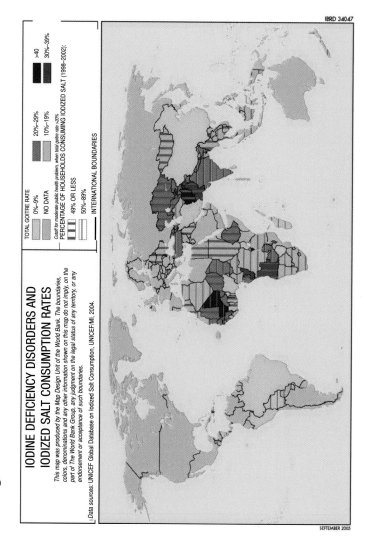

IBRD 34047

IODINE DEFICIENCY DISORDERS AND
IODIZED SALT CONSUMPTION RATES

This map was produced by the Map Design Unit of the World Bank. The boundaries, colors, denominations and any other information shown on this map do not imply, on the part of The World Bank Group, any judgment on the legal status of any territory, or any endorsement or acceptance of such boundaries.

Data sources: UNICEF Global Database on Iodized Salt Consumption, UNICEF/MI, 2004.

TOTAL GOITRE RATE
- 0%–9%
- NO DATA
- 20%–29%
- 10%–19%
- >40
- 30%–39%

Cutoff for moderate public health problem, when total goitre rate >20%
PERCENTAGE OF HOUSEHOLDS CONSUMING IODIZED SALT (1998–2002):
- 49% OR LESS
- 50%–89%
- INTERNATIONAL BOUNDARIES

SEPTEMBER 2005

1
Why Invest in Nutrition?

Improving nutrition contributes to productivity, economic development, and poverty reduction by improving physical work capacity, cognitive development, school performance, and health by reducing disease and mortality. Poor nutrition perpetuates the cycle of poverty and malnutrition through three main routes— direct losses in productivity from poor physical status and losses caused by disease linked with malnutrition; indirect losses from poor cognitive development and losses in schooling; and losses caused by increased health care costs. The economic costs of malnutrition are very high—several billion dollars a year in terms of lost gross domestic product (GDP). Relying on markets and economic growth alone means it will take more than a generation to solve the problem. But specific investments can accelerate improvement, especially programs for micronutrient fortification and supplementation and community-based growth promotion. The economic returns to investing in such programs are very high.

Nutrition and Economics

For many people, the ethical, human rights, and national security arguments for improving nutrition or the tenets of their religious faith are reason enough for action. But there are also strong economic arguments for investing in nutrition:

- Improving nutrition increases productivity and economic growth.
- Not addressing malnutrition has high costs in terms of higher budget outlays as well as lost GDP.
- Returns from programs for improving nutrition far outweigh their costs.

Improved nutrition increases productivity and economic growth

Good nutrition is a basic building block of human capital and, as such, contributes to economic development. In turn, sustainable and equitable growth in developing countries will convert these countries to "developed" states.[1] There is much evidence that nutrition and economic development have a two-way relationship. Improved economic development contributes to improved nutrition (albeit at a very modest pace), but more importantly, improved nutrition drives stronger economic growth. Furthermore, as quantified in the Copenhagen Consensus,[2] productivity losses caused by malnutrition are linked to three kinds of losses—those due to:

- Direct losses in physical productivity.
- Indirect losses from poor cognitive losses and loss in schooling.
- Losses in resources from increased health care costs (figure 1.1).

Therefore, malnutrition hampers both the physical capacity to perform work as well as earning ability.[3]

Malnutrition leads to direct losses in physical productivity

Malnutrition leads to death or disease that in turn reduces productivity. For example:

- According to the World Health Organization (WHO), underweight is the single largest risk factor contributing to the global burden of disease in the developing world. It leads to nearly 15 percent of the total DALY (disability-adjusted life years) losses in countries with high child mortality. In the developed world, overweight is the seventh highest risk factor and it contributes 7.4 percent of DALY losses (technical annex 1.1).[4]
- Malnutrition is directly or indirectly associated with nearly 60 percent of all child mortality[5] and even mildly underweight children have nearly double the risk of death of their well-nourished counterparts.
- Infants with low birthweight (less than 2.5 kilograms)—reflecting, in part, malnutrition in the womb—are at 2 to 10 times the risk of death compared with normal-birthweight infants.[6] These same low-birth-weight infants are at a higher risk of noncommunicable diseases (NCDs) such as diabetes and cardiovascular disease in adulthood.
- Vitamin A deficiency compromises the immune systems of approximately 40 percent of the developing world's children under age five, leading to the deaths of approximately 1 million young children each year.

- Severe iron deficiency anemia causes the deaths in pregnancy and child-birth of more than 60,000 young women a year.
- Iodine deficiency in pregnancy causes almost 18 million babies a year to be born mentally impaired; even mildly or moderately iodine-deficient children have IQs that are 10 to 15 points lower than those not deficient.
- Maternal folate deficiency leads to a quarter of a million severe birth defects every year.[7]

Figure 1.1 The vicious cycle of poverty and malnutrition

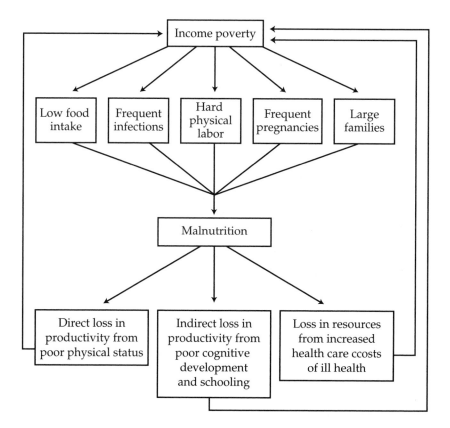

Source: Modified from World Bank (2002a); Bhagwati and others (2004).

The strongest and best documented productivity-nutrition relation-ships are those related to human capital development in early life. Height has unequivocally been shown to be related to productivity,[8] and final height is determined in large part by nutrition from conception to age two. A 1% loss in adult height as a result of childhood stunting is associated with a 1.4 percent loss in productivity.[9] In addition, severe vitamin and mineral deficiencies in the womb and in early childhood can cause blindness, dwarfism, mental retardation, and neural tube defects—all severe handicaps in any society, but particularly limiting in developing countries.

Anemia has a direct and immediate effect on productivity in adults, especially those in physically demanding occupations. Eliminating anemia results in a 5 to 17 percent increase in adult productivity, which adds up to 2 percent of GDP in the worst affected countries.[10] Malnourished adults are also likely to have higher absenteeism because of illness.

In addition to its effect on immune function, poor nutrition also increases susceptibility to chronic diseases in adulthood (see chapter 2). Diet-related NCDs include cardiovascular disease, high blood cholesterol, obesity, adult-onset diabetes, osteoporosis, high blood pressure, and some cancers. About 60 percent of all deaths around the world and 47 percent of the burden of disease can be attributed to diet-related chronic diseases. About two-thirds of deaths linked to these diseases occur in the developing world, where the major risk factors are poor diet, physical inactivity, and obesity.[11] These diseases are increasing at such a rapid rate, even in poor countries, that the phenomenon has been dubbed "the nutrition transition."[12] Like other types of malnutrition, diet-related chronic diseases have their origins in early childhood, often in the womb. They are strongly associated with both low birthweight and stunting in low-income countries.

Strauss and Thomas (1998) have argued through the efficiency wage hypothesis that there is a relationship between calorie intake and work output. Although the hypothesis has yet to be proven, they have shown that calorie intake has an effect on farm output and piece rates of agricultural laborers. They have also shown that in Brazil and in the United States, height and weight of adults (measured as body mass index, or BMI) both affect wages, even after controlling for education. Among low-income men in Brazil, a 1 percent increase in height was associated with a 4 percent increase in wages. The relationship between BMI and productivity decreases as BMI drops below 18.5, showing that adults with extremely low weights (for their heights) have lower productivity. Adults with a high BMI of 24–26 (an indicator of overweight), also have lower productivity. Although the nutrition and productivity relationship is strongest for manual labor, it has also been found in the manufacturing sector and among white collar workers.[13]

Malnutrition leads to indirect losses in productivity from poor cognitive development and schooling. Low birthweight may reduce a person's IQ by 5 percentage points, stunting may reduce it by 5 to 11 points, and iodine deficiency by as much as 10 to 15 points.[14] Iron deficiency anemia consistently reduces performance on tests of mental abilities (including IQ) by 8 points or 0.5 to 1.5 standard deviations in children.[15]

Growth failure before the age of two, anemia during the first two years of life, and iodine deficiency in the womb can have profound and irreversible effects on a child's ability to learn.[16] Malnutrition in Zimbabwe has been calculated to reduce lifetime earnings by 12 percent because of its effect on schooling.[17]

Height and weight affect the likelihood that children will be enrolled at the right time in school. Small and sickly children are often enrolled too late (or never), and they tend to stay in school for less time.[18] Malnutrition also affects the ability to learn. Common sense tells us that a hungry child cannot learn properly. Although this is true and short-term hunger does affect cognitive function (particularly attention span),[19] the effects of immediate hunger pale in comparison with the effects on school performance of malnutrition in early life, long before the child ever reaches the classroom. Children who were malnourished early in life score worse on tests of cognitive function, psychomotor function, and fine motor skills and they have reduced attention spans and lower activity levels.[20] These cognitive skill deficits persist into adulthood and have a direct effect on earnings.[21]

Recent studies have shown that that the positive correlation between nutritional status and both cognitive development and educational attainment also applies to children in normal birthweight and height ranges.[22] For example, as birthweight increased by 100 grams among sibling pairs, the mean IQ at age 7 increased 0.5 point for boys and 0.1 point for girls. Educational attainment at age 26 among cohorts with birthweights between 3 and 3.5 kilograms was 1.4 times higher compared with those with birthweights between 2.5 and 3 kilograms. The odds of having attained higher education (beyond compulsory schooling) at age 26 were also 2.6 times higher among the tallest cohort compared with the shortest cohort.

It is also worth noting here that the effect of improved nutrition often extends into the range of what is considered normal—so that improving birthweights has a positive effect even for children above the 2,500-gram cutoff for low-birthweight babies, reducing anemia has similar benefits beyond those for people afflicted with "severe or moderate" anemia, and levels of mortality are higher even among mildly underweight children.

Not addressing malnutrition has high costs in lost GDP and higher budget outlays

Malnutrition costs low-income countries billions of dollars a year. A recent study, for example, showed that preventing one child from being born with a low birthweight is worth $580.[23, 24] At the country level, it has been estimated that obesity and related NCDs cost China about 2 percent of GDP and in India productivity losses (manual work only) from stunting, iodine deficiency, and iron deficiency together are responsible for a loss of 2.95 percent of GDP.[25, 26]

Preventing micronutrient deficiencies alone in China will be worth between $2.5 and $5 billion annually in increased GDP, which represents 0.2 to 0.4 percent of annual GDP in China. Other studies have suggested that micronutrient deficiencies alone may cost India $2.5 billion annually, about 0.4 percent of India's annual GDP.[27] One estimate suggests that the productivity losses in India associated with undernutrition, iron deficiency anemia, and iodine deficiency disorders (IDD), in the absence of appropriate interventions, will amount to about $114 billion between 2003 and 2012 (India's annual GDP is about $601 billion).[28] Another study, examining only the productivity losses associated with forgone wage employment resulting from child malnutrition, estimates the loss at $2.3 billion in India (0.4 percent of annual GDP). In Sierra Leone, lack of adequate policies and programs to address anemia among women will result in agricultural productivity losses among the female labor force exceeding $94.5 million over the next five years.[29]

Malnourished children require more health services and more expensive types of care than other children. Malnourished children have poorer schooling outcomes and may repeat years more often,[30] thus increasing education costs. Developing countries are also spending an average of 2 to 7 percent of their health care budgets on direct costs for treatment of obesity and associated chronic diseases—and the obesity problem is rapidly worsening (see chapter 2). All of these costs fall largely on governments, which provide extensive public sector financing for health and education for the poor.

Returns from programs for improving nutrition far outweigh their costs

Taking into account the reduced mortality, reduced medical costs, intergenerational benefits (reduced likelihood of giving birth to a low-birthweight infant in the next generation), and increased productivity, Behrman, Alderman, and Hoddinott (2004) calculate that the returns from investing in nutrition are high (table 1.1).

Table 1.1 The benefit-cost ratios for nutrition programs

Intervention programs	Benefit-cost
Breastfeeding promotion in hospitals	5–67
Integrated child care programs	9–16
Iodine supplementation (women)	15–520
Vitamin A supplementation (children < 6 years)	4–43
Iron fortification (per capita)	176–200
Iron supplementation (per pregnant woman)	6–14

Source: Behrman, Alderman, and Hoddinott (2004).

Costs are rarely evaluated rigorously in development programs, and nutrition programs are no exception. Where data have been collected (table 1.2 and annex 1), many nutrition programs are found to be not only effective, but also efficient. For example, eliminating Vitamin A deficiency alone will save 16 percent of the global burden of disease in children.[31] Comparable estimates are available from other sources (table 1.3).

Nutrition, economic growth, and markets

The past 20 years have shown that in many developing countries where incomes have increased substantially, malnutrition has not declined correspondingly. This indicates that economic growth and markets alone are not enough to address malnutrition.

How far can economic growth take us?

The income–malnutrition relationship is modest. When gross national product (GNP) per capita in developing countries doubles, nutrition does improve but the changes in underweight rates are much more modest— from 32 to 23 percent (figure 1.2).

Nutrition has steadily improved in most regions of the developing world—for example, worldwide, stunting fell from 49 to 27 percent of children under age five between 1980 and 2005, and underweight rates declined from 38 to 23 percent between 1980 and 2005 (see chapter 2 and technical annex 1.2). Economic growth has played an important part in this improvement. But economic growth reduces malnutrition very slowly. On the basis of the past correlation between growth and nutrition, it is estimated that sustained per capita economic growth of 2.5 percent between the 1990s and 2015 would reduce malnutrition by 27 percent—only half of the MDG target.[32] Technical annex 1.3 outlines the number of years it would take for different countries to halve their underweight rates at different rates of economic growth. These estimations show that countries cannot depend on economic growth alone to reduce malnutrition within an acceptable timeframe, especially given the human and economic costs and the international community's commitments to achieving the MDGs.

Table 1.2 Annual unit costs of nutrition programs

Intervention	Unit cost per participant ($)
Community-based growth promotion[a]	1.60–10.00 without supplementary food 11.00–18.00 with targeted supplementary feeding
Food supplementation[b]	36.00–172.00 to provide 1,000 Kcal/day
Early child development/child care[c]	250.00–412.00 with food (Bolivia) 2.00–3.00 without food (Uganda)
Nutrition education[d]	2.50
Breastfeeding promotion in hospitals[e]	0.30–0.40 if infant formula removed from maternity 2.00–3.00 if not
Microcredit cum nutrition education[f]	0.90–3.50 (cost of nutrition education only)
Conditional cash transfers[g]	70.00–77.00
Vitamin A supplements to preschool children[h]	1.01–2.55
Vitamin A fortification of sugar[i]	0.69–0.98
Iron supplementation[j]	0.55–3.17
Salt iodization[k]	0.20–0.50

Sources:
a. Fiedler (2003); Iannotti and Gillespie (2002); Gillespie, Mason, and Martorell (1996); Mason and others (2001).
b. Horton (1993, 1999).
c. World Bank (2002a); Alderman (personal communication).
d. Ho (1985).
e. Horton and others (1996).
f. Vor der Bruegge, Dickey, and Dunford (1997; updated 1999).
g. Caldes, Coady, and Maluccio (2004).
h. Fiedler and others (2000); Hendricks, Saitowitz, and Fiedler (1998); Fiedler (2000); Gillespie, Mason, and Martorell (1996).
i. Fiedler (2000); Horton (1999).
j. Horton (1992); Mason and others (2001).
k. Horton (1999); Mason and others (2001).

In Tanzania and India, at realistic levels of sustained per capita GDP (2.1 percent and 3 percent, respectively) and using an elasticity figure (change in malnutrition rates relative to per capita income growth) of -0.5, economic growth alone would take until 2065 and 2035, respectively, to achieve the nutrition MDG (figure 1.3). Depending on income alone, both

Table 1.3 Cost of nutrition interventions ($)

Intervention	Delivery method Fortification	Supplementation
Iodine	0.02–0.05	0.8–2.75[a]
Vitamin A	0.17	0.9–1.25
Iron	0.09–1.00	3.17–5.30
Community-based growth promotion	Less intensive 2.00–5.00	More intensive 5.00–10.00[b]

Source: Caulfield and others (2004b).
a. For iodized oil injections.
b. For example, with paid workers or food supplements.

Figure 1.2 The income–malnutrition relationship

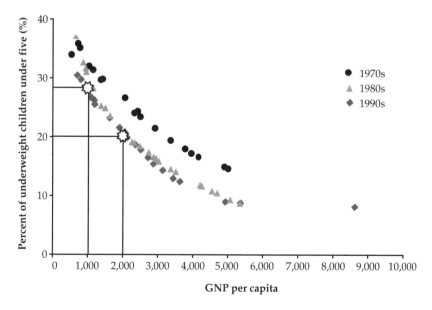

Source: Haddad and others (2002).

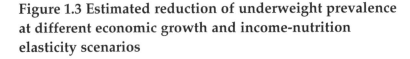

Figure 1.3 Estimated reduction of underweight prevalence at different economic growth and income-nutrition elasticity scenarios

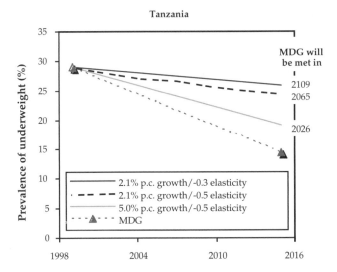

Source: Underweight prevalence in 1999 from www.measuredhs.com. The projections are authors' calculations using different assumptions.

Table 1.4 Reduction of the fraction of children underweight in Tanzania under different income growth and nutrition intervention coverage scenarios (%)

					Reduction in underweight (%)				
Per capita income growth (%) since 1993	Reduction in income poverty (%)	No more interventions	Interventions in 10% more communities	Interventions in 50% more communities	Interventions in all communities	Farm income maximum of 75% of total household income	Additional year of education for the father	Ratio of children vaccinated increased to 95%
0.0	0.0	0.0	11.0	31.7	**53.4**	1.8	3.6	9.9
0.5	24.7	3.4	14.1	34.4	**55.5**	5.2	7.0	12.9
1.0	44.1	6.8	17.2	37.0	**57.6**	8.5	10.3	15.9
1.5	**55.7**	10.1	20.2	39.5	**59.6**	11.8	13.5	18.8
2.0	**66.6**	13.3	23.2	42.0	**61.5**	15.0	16.7	21.7
2.5	**79.0**	16.5	26.0	44.4	**63.4**	18.1	19.7	24.5
3.0	**84.1**	19.5	28.8	46.7	**65.1**	21.1	22.7	27.2

Source: Alderman, Hoogeveen, and Rossi (2005).
Note: Based on data from Kagera district. Simulations are based on the random effect regression model, which is the preferred estimation strategy. Base year is 1993. Because the per capita income growth rate between 1993 and 2003 in Tanzania is known (0.7 percent per year), the effective growth rates required to attain the 1993–2015 mean growth rates of 0, 1, 2, and 3 percent for the 2003–15 period are respectively: –0.5, 1.3, 3.1, and 5.0 percent. Figures in bold show attainment of the MDG.

countries would need an unrealistic sustained rate of per capita income growth of 5.5 percent to achieve the MDG by 2015—unachievable under any circumstances (see technical annex 1.3).

One small study applying data from the Kagera district in Tanzania shows that the income poverty target could be reached with a potentially achievable rate of per capita income growth of 1.5 percent. However, without any nutrition interventions, the corresponding improvement in the nonincome poverty target (nutrition) will be only 10 percent. Even with a per capita income growth of 3 percent, without nutrition interventions, the nutrition MDG cannot be achieved (table 1.4). Near-complete nutrition program coverage is required to achieve the nutrition MDG.

Market forces do not suffice to improve nutrition;
public investment is necessary

Although the private returns of improved nutrition are considerable, malnutrition persists. In part this is due to simple resource constraints that inhibit poor families from investing more resources (which they often do not have and cannot borrow) in children—investments that will not pay off for 10 or 20 years.

A critical reason for market failure in addressing malnutrition has to do with informational asymmetries of two kinds:

* People cannot tell when their children are becoming malnourished because healthy growth rates, arguably the best indicator of good nutrition, cannot be detected with the naked eye. And until micronutrient deficiencies are severe, they are impossible to detect without clinical tests. Thus families do not know there is a nutrition problem until it is too late.
* Good nutrition is not intuitive: people do not always know what food or what feeding practices are best for their children or for themselves. Sometimes, too, food marketing and advertising change preferences in unhealthy ways, as is especially evident in the emerging epidemic of obesity and diet-related NCDs in developing countries, driven by the increased availability of inexpensive, calorie-dense foods.

Because of such information gaps, even when families gain additional cash resources—for example through cash cropping[33] or conditional cash transfers[34]—children's nutrition does not automatically improve. Given the productive and redistributive benefits of investing in nutrition, there is thus an argument for public intervention to ensure that parents get the information they need and to institute policies and programs (such as mandatory salt iodization) that bridge the information gaps.

Yet another reason for justifying public investment is that improved nutrition is often a public good (as opposed to a private good), yielding benefits for everybody in society—for example, better nutrition can reduce the spread of contagious diseases and it increases national economic productivity. Furthermore, the infrastructure and institutions for delivering nutrition services as well as the authority to implement public interventions lie primarily in the public sector, though some interventions (such as food fortification) require much stronger private sector intervention.

Table 1.5 Prevalence of underweight and anemia in Indian children by income quintiles

Income quintiles	*Percentage of children with weight-for-age lower than 2 standard deviations below the mean*			*Percentage of children age 6–59 months with iron levels less than g/dl*
	Male	*Female*	*Both*	*Both*
1992–93 National Family and Health Survey (children 0–3 years)				
Lowest	61.5	60.3	61.0	—
Second	62.5	58.9	60.6	—
Middle	57.1	56.9	57.0	—
Fourth	47.5	49.6	48.5	—
Highest	36.0	35.1	35.6	—
1998–99 National Family and Health Survey (children 0–2 years)				
Lowest	59.7	61.5	60.7	78.8
Second	51.7	56.5	54.0	79.0
Middle	47.2	51.3	49.2	75.1
Fourth	37.6	40.3	38.9	72.3
Highest	25.2	27.6	26.4	63.9

Source: Gwatkin and others (2003).
— = not available.

Nutrition and income poverty

Undernutrition and micronutrient malnutrition are themselves direct indicators of poverty, in the broader definition of the term that includes human development. But undernutrition is also strongly linked to income poverty, although by no means synonymous with it. The prevalence of malnutrition is often two or three times—and sometimes many times—higher among the poorest income quintile than among the highest quintile.[35] (Table 1.5 illustrates the situation in India, which has almost 40 percent of the world's malnourished children.[36]) This means that improving nutrition is pro-poor and increases the income-earning potential of the poor. In countries where girls' nutrition lags behind, improving the nutrition of young girls adds an extra equity-enhancing dimension to any such investment.

Poverty and malnutrition reinforce each other through a vicious cycle (see figure 1.1). Poverty is associated with poor diets, unhealthy environments, physically demanding labor, and high fertility, which increase malnutrition (chapter 2). Malnutrition in turn reduces health, education, and immediate and future income, thus perpetuating poverty. Even worse, poor malnourished women are likely to give birth to low-birthweight babies, thus perpetuating poverty in the subsequent generation. Addressing malnutrition helps break this vicious cycle and stop the intergenerational transmission of poverty and malnutrition.

Nutrition and the Millenium Development Goals

Malnutrition is one of the most important constraints to achieving the MDGs. Improving nutrition is essential to reduce extreme poverty. Recognition of this requirement is evident in the definition of the first MDG, which aims to eradicate extreme poverty and hunger. The two targets are to be halved between 1990 and 2015:

- The proportion of people whose income is less than $1 a day.
- The proportion of people who suffer from hunger (as measured by the percentage of children under age five who are underweight).

The first target refers to income poverty; the second addresses nonincome poverty. The two indicators used for measuring progress on the nonincome poverty goal are:

Box 1.1 Off track on the Millennium Development Goals

Recently the World Bank issued a Global Monitoring Report painting a pessimistic picture for achieving the MDGs on hunger: five years after the global commitment was made, progress has been inadequate to ensure their attainment. Sub-Saharan Africa is not on track to achieve a single MDG. In addition to other goals, it is off track on the hunger goal—and it is the only region where child malnutrition is not declining. South Asia is off track on six goals: gender equity, universal primary school completion, child mortality, maternal mortality, communicable diseases, and sanitation. And while malnutrition in that region is dropping sufficiently to achieve the MDG target, it remains at very high absolute levels: almost half of children under age five are underweight. The Middle East and North Africa is also off track on six goals: gender equity, universal primary completion, child mortality, communicable diseases, water, and sanitation. Europe and Central Asia is off track on child mortality, maternal mortality, communicable diseases, and sanitation. And both Latin America and the Caribbean and East Asia and the Pacific are off track on child mortality, maternal mortality, and communicable diseases.

Source: Excerpted from World Bank (2005b).

Figure 1.4 Progress toward the nonincome poverty target

On track (24%)		Deteriorating status (18%)	
AFR (7)	**LAC (10)**	**AFR (13)**	**ECA (4)**
Angola	Bolivia	Niger	Albania
Benin	Chile	Burkina Faso	Azerbaijan
Botswana	Colombia	Cameroon	Russian Federation
Chad	Dominican Rep.	Comoros	Serbia and Montenegro
Gambia, The	Guyana	Ethiopia	
Mauritania	Haiti	Guinea	**LAC (3)**
Zimbabwe	Jamaica	Lesotho	Argentina
	Mexico	Mali	Costa Rica
EAP (5)	Peru	Senegal*	Panama
China	Venezuela, R.B. de	Sudan	
Indonesia		Tanzania*	**MENA (2)**
Malaysia	**MENA (6)**	Togo	Iraq
Thailand	Algeria	Zambia	Yemen, Rep. of
Vietnam	Egypt, Arab Rep. of		
	Iran, Islamic	**EAP (2)**	**SAR (2)**
ECA (6)	Rep. of Jordan	Mongolia	Maldives
Armenia	Syrian Arab Rep.	Myanmar	Nepal
Croatia	Tunisia		
Kazakhstan			
Kyrgyz Rep.	**SAR (0)**		
Romania		**No trend data available (40%)**	
Turkey			

	AFR (13)	Georgia
	Burundi	Hungary
	Cape Verde	Latvia
Some improvement, but not on track	Congo, Rep. of	Lithuania
	Equatorial Guinea	Macedonia, FYR
AFR (14)	Guinea	Moldova
Central African Rep.	**ECA (0)**	Guinea-Bissau	Poland
Congo, DR		Liberia	Slovak Republic
Côte d'Ivoire	**LAC (4)**	Mauritius	Tajikistan
Eritrea	El Salvador	Namibia	Turkmenistan
Gabon	Guatemala	São Tomé and Principe	Ukraine
Ghana	Honduras	Seychelles	Uzbekistan
Kenya	Nicaragua	Somalia	
Madagascar		South Africa	**LAC (12)**
Malawi	**MENA (1)**	Swaziland	Belize
Mozambique	Morocco		Brazil
Nigeria		**EAP (11)**	Dominica
Rwanda	**SAR (4)**	Fiji	Ecuador
Sierra Leone	Bangladesh*	Kiribati	Grenada
Uganda	India	Marshall Is.	Paraguay
	Pakistan	Micronesia, Federated	St. Kitts and Nevis
EAP (5)	Sri Lanka	States of	St. Lucia
Cambodia		Palau	St. Vincent
Lao PDR		Papua New Guinea	Suriname
Phillippines		Samoa	Trinidad and Tobago
		Solomon Islands	Uruguay
		Timor-Leste	
		Tonga	**MENA (2)**
		Vanuatu	Djibouti
			Lebanon
		ECA (17)	
		Belarus	**SAR (2)**
		Bosnia and	Afghanistan
		Herzegovina	Bhutan
		Bulgaria	
		Czech Republic	
		Estonia	

Source: Author's calculations. See also technical annex 5.6.
Note: All calculations are based on 1990–2002 trend data from the WHO Global Database on Child Growth and Malnutrition (as of April 2005). Countries indicated by an asterisk subsequently released preliminary DHS data that suggest improvement and therefore may be reclassified when their data are officially released.

Figure 1.5 Progress toward the nonincome poverty target (nutrition MDG)

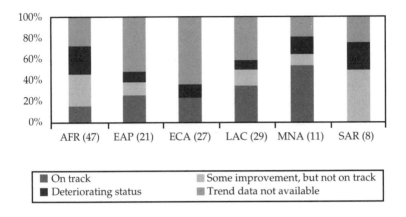

Source: Author's calculations. See also technical annex 5.6.

- The prevalence of underweight children (under age five)
- The proportion of the population consuming less than the minimum level of dietary energy.

Therefore, improving nutrition is in itself an MDG target. Yet most assessments of progress toward the MDGs have focused primarily on the income poverty target, and the prognosis in general is that most countries are on track for achieving the poverty goal. Yet many regions are off track for achieving the nonincome poverty target (box 1.1).

Of 143 countries, only 34 (24 percent) are on track to achieve the nonincome target (nutrition MDG) (figures 1.4 and 1.5). It is particularly notable that no country in South Asia, where undernutrition is the highest, will achieve the MDG—though Bangladesh will come close to achieving it, and Asia as a whole will achieve it. Another alarming note is struck by the many countries where the nutrition status is deteriorating. Many are in Africa, where the nexus between HIV and undernutrition is particularly strong and mutually reinforcing. And in 57 countries, no data are available to tell whether progress is being made.

Improving nutrition is not only intrinsic to achieving the first MDG, but also fundamental to progress toward five other goals (table 1.6).

Nutrition and Human Rights

The 1948 Universal Declaration of Human Rights established adequate health, including adequate food, as a basic human right. The right to health and nutrition was reiterated in the 1989 Convention on the Rights of the Child, adopted by all but two United Nations (UN) member countries. The right to adequate nutrition is also enshrined in the constitutions of many countries—for example, those of Ethiopia, Guatemala, India, Peru, and South Africa. Governments are entrusted to ensure that these rights are fulfilled, especially among children, the elderly, the vulnerable, and the infirm. The rights-based approach to development has also been firmly endorsed by the development community in recent years.

Nutrition interventions also often act as social safety nets against shocks (see box 3.2). This is also true in countries undergoing reforms; access to safety nets such as nutrition interventions can increase the tolerance for shocks from public sector reforms, thereby increasing the potential for the success of reforms while also protecting basic human rights.

The Know-How for Improving Nutrition

As documented by the Copenhagen Consensus, we know what to do to improve nutrition and the expected rates of returns from investing in nutrition are high. Compared with many possible development investments, including trade reform and private sector deregulation, malaria eradication, and water and sanitation, the provision of micronutrients was identified as the second best opportunity for meeting the world's development challenges. Other nutrition investments also ranked high (table 1.7). Direct actions to improve nutrition are therefore desirable and have high potential for returns.

The final argument for investing in nutrition is that there are tried and tested models and experiences for reducing most forms of malnutrition—models and experience that have not been adequately exploited and scaled up (see chapter 4). In some exceptional countries, nutrition programs have virtually universal coverage (Chile, Costa Rica, Cuba, and Thailand) and malnutrition has declined rapidly (see figure 2.12). But other countries with large nutrition programs still have significant gaps in coverage and quality. The reason undernutrition and micronutrient malnutrition persist at high levels is not that we do not know how to reduce them, nor that countries have applied best practice, yet failed to succeed. It is that most

countries have not invested at a scale large enough to get these tested technologies to those who will benefit from them most. In addition, many
countries that have invested have either used less effective and less strategic interventions (such as school feeding), or have not paid attention to
implementation quality.

Table 1.6 How investing in nutrition is critical to achieving the MDGs

Goal	Nutrition effect
Goal 1: Eradicate extreme poverty and hunger.	Malnutrition erodes human capital through irreversible and intergenerational effects on cognitive and physical development.
Goal 2: Achieve universal primary education.	Malnutrition affects the chances that a child will go to school, stay in school, and perform well.
Goal 3: Promote gender equality and empower women.	Antifemale biases in access to food, health, and care resources may result in malnutrition, possibly reducing women's access to assets. Addressing malnutrition empowers women more than men.
Goal 4: Reduce child mortality.	Malnutrition is directly or indirectly associated with most child deaths, and it is the main contributor to the burden of disease in the developing world.
Goal 5: Improve maternal health.	Maternal health is compromised by malnutrition, which is associated with most major risk factors for maternal mortality. Maternal stunting and iron and iodine deficiencies particularly pose serious problems.
Goal 6: Combat HIV/AIDS, malaria, and other diseases.	Malnutrition may increase risk of HIV transmission, compromise antiretroviral therapy, and hasten the onset of full-blown AIDS and premature death. It increases the chances of tuberculosis infection, resulting in disease, and it also reduces malarial survival rates.

Source: Adapted from Gillespie and Haddad (2003).

Table 1.7 The Copenhagen Consensus ranks the provision of micronutrients as a top investment

Rating	Challenge	Opportunity
Very good	1. Diseases 2. Malnutrition and hunger 3. Subsidies and trade 4. Diseases	Controlling HIV/AIDS Providing micronutrients Liberalizing trade Controlling malaria
Good	5. Malnutrition and hunger 6. Sanitation and water 7. Sanitation and water 8. Sanitation and water 9. Government	Developing new agricultural technologies Developing small-scale water technologies Implementing community-managed systems Conducting research on water in agriculture Lowering costs of new business
Fair	10. Migration 11. Malnutrition and hunger 12. Diseases 13. Malnutrition and hunger	Lowering barriers to migration Improving infant and child malutrition Scaling up basic health services Reducing the prevalence of low birthweight
Poor	14–17. Climate/migration	Various

Source: Bhagwati and others (2004).

Table 1.8 Coverage of nutrition interventions in some large-scale programs

Program/country	Coverage rates
ICDS/India	Purported to cover 90% of development blocks, but only half the villages from the lowest two wealth deciles have access to the program, and the individuals not reached seem to be the poorer and younger children[a]
NNP/Bangladesh	Aims to cover 105 of the 464 *upazilas* (< 25% coverage)
AIN/Honduras	Reaches only 24 of 47 health areas
SEECALINE/Madagascar	Reaches only 62 of 111 districts

Source: Various unpublished World Bank reports.
a. Gragnolati and others (forthcoming).

Some program coverage data can be illustrative as a proxy measure of underinvestment compared with the severity of undernutrition (table 1.8 and maps 1.1 and 1.2). While coverage for micronutrients is somewhat higher, similar discrepancies between needs and investments exist (vitamin A and iodine, maps 1.3 and 1.4).

The conclusion: there is a significant gap between the size of the nutrition problem (chapter 2) and the coverage of current investments. Coverage of micronutrient programs is wider than for underweight programs. Nonetheless, investments in both are much smaller than warranted, although many models for and successful experiences in addressing malnutrition exist (chapters 3 and 4).

Notes

1. Hunt (2005).

2. Behrman, Alderman, and Hoddinott (2004).

3. Hunt (2005).

4. Ezzati and others (2002).

5. Pelletier, Frongillo, and Habicht (1994); Caulfield and others (2004a); Caulfield, Richard, and Black (2004); Bryce and others (2005).

6. Behrman, Alderman, and Hoddinott (2004).

7. UNICEF and MI (2004a).

8. Behrman and Rosenzweig (2001).

9. Hunt (2005)

10. Strauss and Thomas (1998); Horton and Ross (2003).

11. IASO (2004).

12. Popkin, Horton, and Kim (2001).

13. Strauss and Thomas (1998).

14. Grantham-McGregor, Fernald, and Sethurahman (1999)

15. Horton and Ross (2003).

16. Behrman, Alderman, and Hoddinott (2004).

17. Behrman, Alderman, and Hoddinott (2004).

18. Behrman, Alderman, and Hoddinott (2004).

19. Pollitt (1990).

20. Behrman, Alderman, and Hoddinott (2004); Pollitt (1990).

21. Behrman, Alderman, and Hoddinott (2004).

22. Richards and others (2001); Richards and others (2002), Matte and others (2001).

23. It was calculated under the assumption that all non-low-birthweight children would survive to adulthood and become laborers. When corrected for age-specific mortality, the benefit becomes $510 (personal communication, Alderman).

24. Alderman and Behrman (2004).

25. IFPRI (2003).

26. Horton (1999).
27. Gragnolati (forthcoming).
28. AED (2003).
29. Darnton-Hill (2005).
30. Behrman, Alderman, and Hoddinott (2004).
31. Darnton-Hill (2005)
32. Haddad (2003).
33. Von Braun (1995).
34. Behrman and Hoddinott (2001); Morris and others (2004).
35. Wagstaff and Watanabe (2001); Gwatkin and others (2003).
36. See Gwatkin and others (2003) for other countries.

2
How Serious Is Malnutrition and Why Does It Happen?

Chapter 1 outlined the economic and other reasons for investing in nutrition. This chapter details the enormous size and scope of the nutrition problem (both underweight and overweight) at global, regional, and country levels to further strengthen the case for investing in nutrition.

Nearly one-third of the world's children are either underweight or stunted, and micronutrient deficiencies affect more than 30 percent of the developing world's population. The poor are the most affected. The malnutrition divide between the developed and the developing world is very wide, and inequities are increasing. Asia continues to have both the highest rates and the largest numbers of malnourished children in the world. Africa is the only continent seeing an increasing rate of undernutrition. The epidemic of obesity and diet-related noncommunicable diseases (NCDs) is emerging in the same countries and often in the same households where undernutrition is already a serious problem.

Evidence shows that malnutrition is not simply a result of household food insecurity: many children in food-secure households are still underweight or stunted because of inappropriate infant feeding and care practices, poor access to health services, or poor sanitation, except under famine conditions. Malnutrition is often linked to gender issues such as women's lack of time. Though malnutrition is higher among the income poor, it also affects the better off—suggesting that behavior is often an underlying cause of malnutrition.

The worst damage from malnutrition takes place from conception through the first two years of life, and most of this early damage is irreversible. Initial evidence suggests that the origins of obesity and diet-related NCDs may also lie in early childhood. Therefore, the best window of opportunity for addressing malnutrition is very small, from before conception through the first two years of age. Later investments and actions are unlikely to be able to reverse the damage from early years.

Over one-fourth of all children in developing countries are either underweight or stunted. One-third of the world's population (almost 2 billion people) suffers from various forms of iodine deficiency disorders (IDD). The same numbers have iron deficiency, which leads to anemia. About a quarter of the children under age five (127 million) suffer from vitamin A deficiency, which increases the risk of early death.[1] Simultaneously, the proportion of people who are overweight or obese is growing, often in the same countries where undernutrition and micronutrient malnutrition are concentrated, leading to what is often referred to as the "double burden of malnutrition." Some 1.1 billion adults are overweight, and 300 million are obese.[2]

Undernutrition

The "malnutrition divide" between the developed and the developing countries is huge. Twenty-seven percent (more than 147 million) of children under age five are stunted and 23 percent (more than 126 million) are underweight in developing countries. Comparable figures for the developed world are 2.6 percent for stunting and 1.1 percent for underweight. In Africa, about 24 percent of children are underweight and 35 percent are stunted; between 35 million and 50 million children under age five are affected. Less well known is that in Asia, average underweight rates are somewhat higher than in Africa (26 percent), and in several large South Asian countries, both underweight and stunting rates are nearly double those in Africa (38 to 51 percent). Undernutrition is therefore worst in Asia, which has 92 million stunted and 89 million underweight children (box 2.1).[3]

In a recent World Health Organization (WHO) study, underweight prevalence in developing countries was forecast to decline by 36 percent (from 30 percent in 1990 to 19 percent in 2015)—significantly below the 50 percent required to meet the MDG over the same time frame.[4] These global data mask interregional differences that are widening disturbingly. Much of the forecast global improvement derives from a projected prevalence decline from 35 to 18 percent in Asia—driven primarily by the improvements in China. By contrast, in Africa, the prevalence is projected to increase from 24 to 27 percent. And the situation in Eastern Africa—a region blighted by HIV/AIDS, which has major interactions with malnutrition—is critical. Here underweight prevalences are forecast to be 25 percent higher in 2015 than they were in 1990.

Even in East Asia, Latin America, and Eastern Europe, many countries continue to carry heavy burdens of undernutrition and micronutrient malnutrition (Cambodia, Indonesia, Lao PDR, the Philippines, and Vietnam; Guatemala, Haiti, and Honduras; and Uzbekistan, to name only a few). In many, such as Guatemala and the Republic of Yemen, the undernutrition

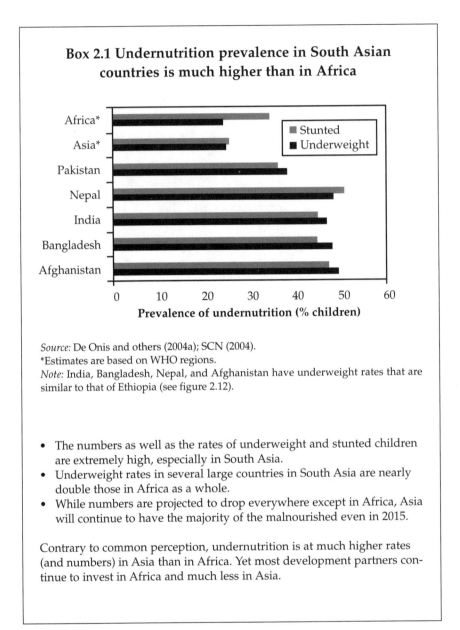

Box 2.1 Undernutrition prevalence in South Asian
countries is much higher than in Africa

Source: De Onis and others (2004a); SCN (2004).
*Estimates are based on WHO regions.
Note: India, Bangladesh, Nepal, and Afghanistan have underweight rates that are
similar to that of Ethiopia (see figure 2.12).

- The numbers as well as the rates of underweight and stunted children
  are extremely high, especially in South Asia.
- Underweight rates in several large countries in South Asia are nearly
  double those in Africa as a whole.
- While numbers are projected to drop everywhere except in Africa, Asia
  will continue to have the majority of the malnourished even in 2015.

Contrary to common perception, undernutrition is at much higher rates
(and numbers) in Asia than in Africa. Yet most development partners continue to invest in Africa and much less in Asia.

rates are well above those in that region as a whole. Chances are that these
high undernutrition rates will escape the attention of the international
development partners unless special efforts are made to highlight this issue
within regions that are doing well at an aggregate level (figure 2.1).

Figure 2.1 Prevalence of and trends in malnutrition among children under age five, 1980–2005

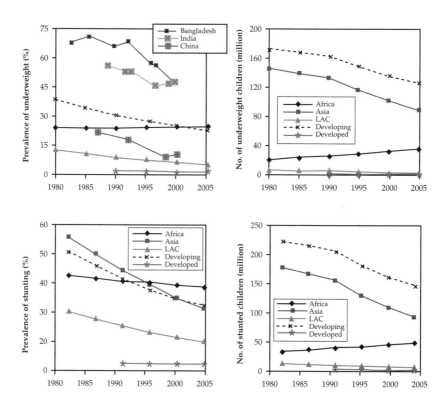

Source: De Onis (2004a); SCN (2004).
Note: Estimates are based on WHO regions. Prevalence and numbers also appear in technical annex 2.1.

Regional and subregional data also mask other inequalities, as evident from the very high rates of underweight in Bangladesh and India (see box 2.1) and the very high rates of undernutrition in countries in Latin America (such as Guatemala), the Middle East and North Africa (such as the Republic of Yemen), and Eastern Europe and Central Asia (such as Uzbekistan) (figure 2.12). Although current trends suggest that Asia may approach the MDG target, wide disparities are likely to remain among Asian countries, with some of the largest countries lagging behind. Inequities are likely to be much larger within these countries—with rural areas, the poorest, and in some cases girls, lagging furthest behind. In absolute numbers, the global total of underweight children is projected to decline by nearly one-third, from 164 million in 1990 to 113 million in 2015.[5] Although numbers are projected to drop everywhere except in Africa, Asia will continue to house the majority of the malnourished in 2015 (figure 2.2).

Inequities in nutrition, including urban-rural differences and income and gender inequities, not only will persist, but often will become larger. Data from India illustrate these inequities across income quintiles for both underweight and anemia rates (see table 1.5). Underweight rates are much higher among the poorest quintile and the rate of decline is much lower, so that over time these inequities between the rich and the poor are widening. Regional and country-specific data on child underweight and stunting prevalence show wide disparities, even across countries in the same regions (figure 2.12 and technical annex 5.6).

Low Birthweight

South Asia has the highest rate of babies born with low birthweight (28 percent), followed by the Middle East and North Africa and the rest of the Africa region. Low birthweight is much less of a problem in Latin America and the Caribbean, East Asia and the Pacific, and Europe and

Figure 2.2 Projected trends in numbers of underweight children under age five, 1990–2015

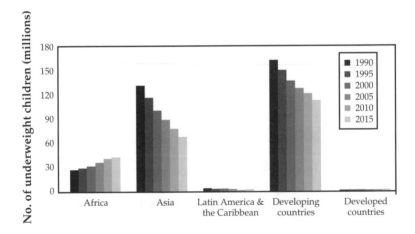

Source: De Onis and others (2004a, 2004b).
Note: Estimates are based on WHO regions.

Central Asia. High rates of low birthweight contribute to the high rates of underweight and stunting, especially in South Asia. The large population in South Asia means that this rate is multiplied several times over—so that South Asia has the highest number of babies born with low weights, setting the stage for having the largest numbers of undernourished children. Birthweight is an issue in Africa as well, but on a smaller scale.

Figure 2.3 Prevalence and number of low-birthweight infants

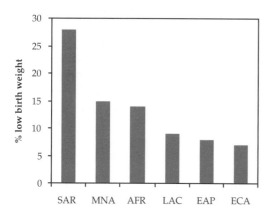

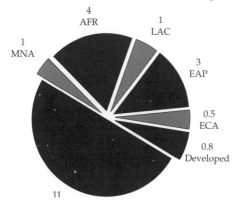

Millions of children born with low birthweight

Source: UNICEF and WHO (2004).
Note: Estimates are based on UNICEF regions.

Low-birthweight children are disadvantaged even before they are born, and evidence suggests that these children rarely catch up in growth.[6] Furthermore, data suggest that the major causes of low birthweight are poor maternal nutrition, anemia, malaria, diarrhea, sexually transmitted diseases, and diseases, such as schistosomiasis, where they are endemic. In more industrial countries, cigarette smoking during pregnancy is the leading cause of low birthweight.[7]

Recent research has shown that babies born with low birthweight are much more prone to abdominal obesity and noncommunicable diseases in adult life. This phenomenon, referred to as the "Barker hypothesis" or "the fetal origins of adult disease," is still being debated, primarily because most evidence supporting the hypothesis comes from observational rather than experimental settings.[8] We do not aim to review the entire literature here, simply to note that evidence to support this hypothesis has been documented in varied observational settings in the developed and developing world (the Netherlands, Sweden, India, China, and several other countries).[9] In Japan, results from one study suggest that lower birthweight and lower rate of height increase during childhood are independently associated with increases in blood pressure and serum cholesterol in adult life.[10] In Finland, low birthweights for height have been shown to be associated with increased risk of coronary heart disease, and low height and weight at age one year also increased the risk.[11]

Data from longitudinal studies on 300,000 19-year-old conscripts exposed to the Dutch famine of 1944–45 show that maternal malnutrition during early pregnancy was associated with higher body mass index (BMI, weight for height) and waist circumference in 50-year-old women, but not in men. The analyses also showed that the rate of obesity was higher in women who had been exposed to famine in early pregnancy, as compared with those exposed to famine in the last trimester.[12] The timing of the food deprivation (early or later in pregnancy) also determined susceptibility to diabetes and high blood pressure.[13]

Many of these observational studies conclude that improvements in fetal, infant, and child growth could substantially reduce the incidence of NCDs in adulthood. This link could explain why the same developing countries that have high numbers of low-birthweight and underweight children are now experiencing the double burden of increasing numbers of adults who are overweight or have NCDs, as documented in the following sections.

Obesity and Diet-Related Noncommunicable Diseases

The International Obesity Task Force estimates that about 1.1 billion adults are overweight, including more than 300 million who are obese.[14] Childhood overweight affects about 155 million school-age children, including about 40 million who are obese. Overweight and NCDs account for about 46 percent of the global burden of disease and about 60 percent of total global deaths, 79 percent of which occur in developing countries.[15] The attributable mortality and burden of disease are expected to grow to 73 percent and 60 percent by 2020. Trends in overnutrition rates—observed as obesity or as an excess of added sugar and saturated or trans-fatty acids in the diet—are alarming. Take three examples from three continents: In Mexico, rates of adult male obesity have tripled since 1988; in China, more than 200 million adults are affected—a 2002 survey revealed national adult overweight at 23 percent, obesity at 7 percent, and childhood obesity at more than 8 percent; in South Africa in 1998, 29 percent of men and 56 percent of women were overweight or obese.[16] High rates of overweight increasingly coexist with high rates of underweight—a 1999 national survey in China found one in five overweight children under age 9 had suffered from stunting because of chronic undernutrition early in life.

Trends in overweight among children under age five, though based on data from a limited number of countries, are alarming (figure 2.4)—for all developing countries and particularly for those in Africa, where rates seem to be increasing at a far greater rate (58 percent increase) than in the developing world as a whole (17 percent increase). The lack of data prevents definitive answers for why Africa is experiencing this exaggerated trend; however, the correlation between maternal overweight and child overweight suggests that one of the answers may lie therein (figure 2.5).

Comparable data for overweight and obesity rates among mothers show similar alarming trends. Countries in the Middle East and North Africa have the highest maternal overweight rates, followed by those in Latin America and the Caribbean. However, several African countries have more than 20 percent maternal overweight rates—in Mauritania, more than 40 percent of mothers are overweight.

Also evident is that overweight coexists in the same countries where both child and maternal undernutrition are very widespread and in many countries with low per capita GNP (figures 2.6 and 2.7). Furthermore, as many as 60 percent of households with an underweight person also had an overweight person, demonstrating that underweight and overweight coexist not only in the same countries, but also in the same households.[17] Again, these data support the premise that access to and availability of food at the household level are not the major causes of undernutrition.

Figure 2.4 Trends in obesity among children under age five

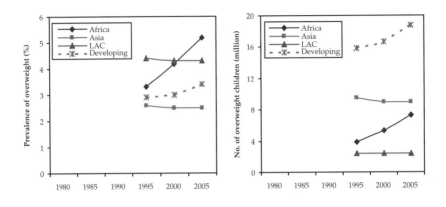

Source: SCN (2004).
Note: Estimates are based on WHO regions.

Figure 2.5 Maternal and child overweight

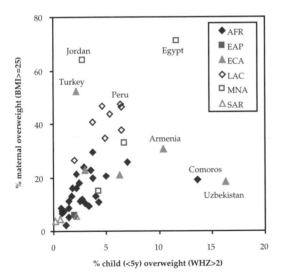

Source: Author's calculations using data from measuredhs.com.

Figure 2.6 Maternal overweight versus maternal and child undernutrition

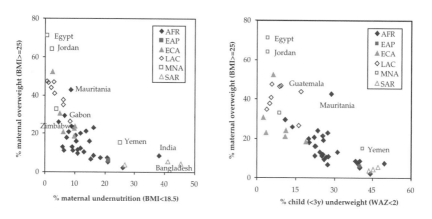

Source: Author's calculations using data from measuredhs.com.

Figure 2.7 Coexistence of energy deficiency and obesity in low- and middle-income countries

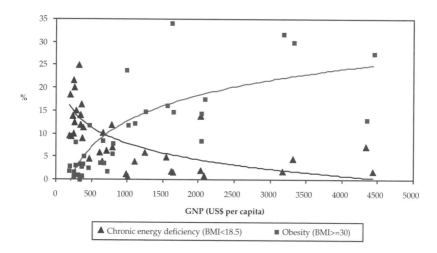

Source: Monteiro and others (2004).

Micronutrient Malnutrition

Deficiencies of key vitamins and minerals continue to be pervasive and they overlap considerably with problems of general undernutrition (underweight and stunting). A recent global progress report states that 35 percent of people in the world lack adequate iodine, 40 percent of people in the developing world suffer from iron deficiency, and more than 40 percent of children are vitamin A deficient (figures 2.8 and 2.9).[18] In summary, the scale of the malnutrition problem is very large and, given its consequences for economic development, calls for immediate and large-scale action.

Figure 2.8 Prevalence of subclinical vitamin A deficiency in children age 0–72 months, by region, 1990–2000

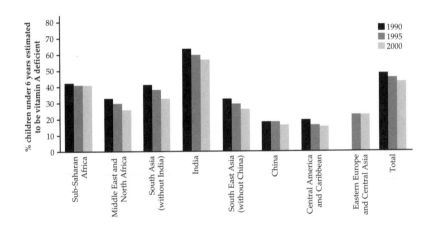

Source: UNICEF and MI (2004b).
Note: Estimates are based on UNICEF regions.

Figure 2.9 Prevalence of iron deficiency in preschool children, by region, 1990–2000

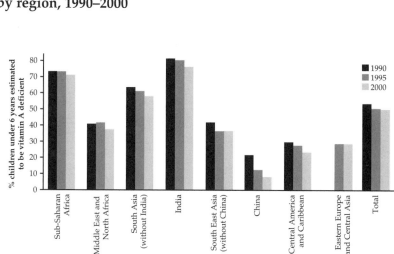

Source: UNICEF and MI (2004).
Note: Estimates are based on UNICEF regions.

What Causes Malnutrition, and Who Is Worst Affected?

At an immediate level, an individual becomes malnourished because of inadequate or inappropriate dietary intake, ill health, or both. These two factors often interact in a negative synergy. Illness reduces appetite and increases nutrient requirements, while inadequate intake of food (quantity or quality) makes the body more susceptible to illness. Underlying this vicious cycle are household or community deficits in food security, inadequate access to health and environmental services, and household childcare behaviors and practices. These three underlying factors—often summarized as "food, health, and care"—also interact, and they too are underpinned by more basic causes relating to the amount, control, and use of resources and capacity in societies.[19]

Undernutrition is often assumed to result primarily from food insecurity, but data from many countries suggest that food is not the only and often not even the main cause of undernutrition, except under famine conditions. Data show that at any given level of food availability, underweight rates can range from as low as 2 to 10 percent to as high as 40 to 70 percent

Figure 2.10 Prevalence of underweight children by per capita dietary energy supply, by region, 1970–96

Percent of underweight children under age five

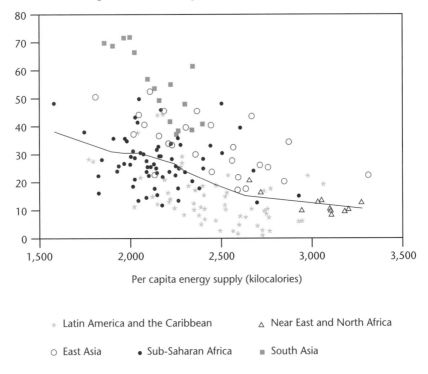

Per capita energy supply (kilocalories)

✳ Latin America and the Caribbean	△ Near East and North Africa
○ East Asia • Sub-Saharan Africa	▪ South Asia

Source: Haddad and Smith (1999).

(figure 2.10). The conclusion, confirmed by many studies,[20] is not that food supplies are irrelevant, but that other factors, such as maternal knowledge, caring practices for young children, access to health services, and water and sanitation, have important roles to play. Data from many countries show high undernutrition rates in regions and households where food is plentiful: examples are the Arsi region in Ethiopia and the Iringa region in Tanzania, both of which have high food production rates yet also very high stunting rates—62 percent in Arsi and 66 percent in Iringa.[21]

Other data also show that higher agricultural production and higher income do not guarantee improved nutrition. Although the nutritional

Undernutrition is not just a state, but a process whose consequences often extend not only into later life, but also into future generations. The process often starts in the womb (especially in South Asia), and continues through at least the first two years of life (box 2.2). The critical periods of pregnancy and lactation and the first two years of life pose special nutritional challenges because these are when nutrition requirements are greatest and when these population subgroups, in many parts of the world, are most vulnerable to inadequate caring behaviors, inadequate access to health services, and inappropriate feeding practices.

Pregnancy and lactation substantially increase nutritional needs to support adequate fetal growth and breastfeeding, and the additional energy and nutrient demands easily place pregnant and lactating women at great nutritional risk. When pregnancies occur during the teenage years, the risk is even higher because of the competition for nutritional requirements between the mother's needs and the babies' needs—that is, between the mother's preparation for lactation and the fetal growth and development.[23] Children of adolescent mothers are also often at greater risk of poor nutritional care and feeding practices. Therefore women need access to appropriate health care and nutrition information as well as appropriate foods during pregnancy and lactation more than during any other period.

Very young children are the most susceptible to infections. They need the dietary inputs (through exclusive breastfeeding and timely complementary feeding) to support the fast rate of growth that typically occurs in the first two years of life. They are the least able to make their needs known

Figure 2.11 Prevalence of overweight among children under age five, by age group

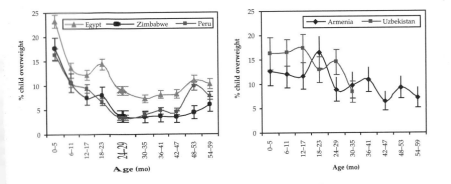

Source: Data from measuredhs.com; authors' calculations.

status of children from the richest 20 percent of households is much b
than that of children from the poorest 20 percent in many countries
example, the Dominican Republic, Morocco, Nicaragua, Peru, and Turk
the proportion of underweight children does not differ much by inco
level in many other countries (for example, Burkina Faso, Cambo
Ethiopia, Kazakhstan, Madagascar, Niger, Tanzania, and Turkmenistan
In India (as in many other countries), even among the richest quintile,
percent of preschool children are underweight and 64 percent are anen
(see table 1.5), showing that food insecurity and poverty are not the on
causes of undernutrition.

Box 2.2 The window of opportunity for addressing undernutrition

The window of opportunity for improving nutrition is small—from
pre-pregnancy through the first two years of life. There is consensus that
the damage to physical growth, brain development, and human capital
formation that occurs during this period is extensive and largely irreversible. Therefore interventions must focus on this window of opportunity. Any investments after this critical period are much less likely to
improve nutrition.

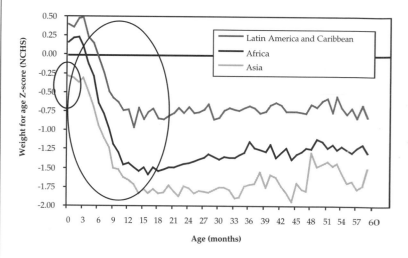

Source: Shrimpton and others (2001).
Note: Estimates are based on WHO regions.

and the most vulnerable to the effects of poor care practices. In fact, the main causes of the often precipitous decline in nutritional status immediately after birth (see box 2.2) are often inadequate feeding and caring practices rather than a lack of food in the household. Data also show that the damage done by undernutrition very early in life, to both physical growth and brain development, is largely irreversible.[24]

Box 2.3 Three myths about nutrition

Poor nutrition is implicated in more than half of all child deaths worldwide—a proportion unmatched by any infectious disease since the Black Death. It is intimately linked with poor health and environmental factors. But planners, politicians, and economists often fail to recognize these connections. Serious misapprehensions include the following myths:

Myth 1: *Malnutrition is primarily a matter of inadequate food intake.* Not so. Food is of course important. But most serious malnutrition is caused by bad sanitation and disease, leading to diarrhea, especially among young children. Women's status and women's education play big parts in improving nutrition. Improving care of young children is vital.

Myth 2: *Improved nutrition is a by-product of other measures of poverty reduction and economic advance. It is not possible to jump-start the process.* Again, untrue. Improving nutrition requires focused action by parents and communities, backed by local and national action in health and public services, especially water and sanitation. Thailand has shown that moderate and severe malnutrition can be reduced by 75 percent or more in a decade by such means.

Myth 3: *Given scarce resources, broad-based action on nutrition is hardly feasible on a mass scale, especially in poor countries.* Wrong again. In spite of severe economic setbacks, many developing countries have made impressive progress. More than two-thirds of the people in developing countries now eat iodized salt, combating the iodine deficiency and anemia that affect about 3.5 billion people, especially women and children in some 100 nations. About 450 million children a year now receive vitamin A capsules, tackling the deficiency that causes blindness and increases child mortality. New ways have been found to promote and support breastfeeding, and breastfeeding rates are being maintained in many countries and increased in some. Mass immunization and promotion of oral rehydration to reduce deaths from diarrhea have also done much to improve nutrition.

Source: Extracted from Jolly (1996).

Figure 2.12 Underweight prevalence and rates of decline in World Bank regions and countries

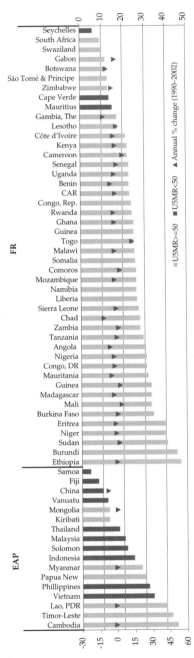

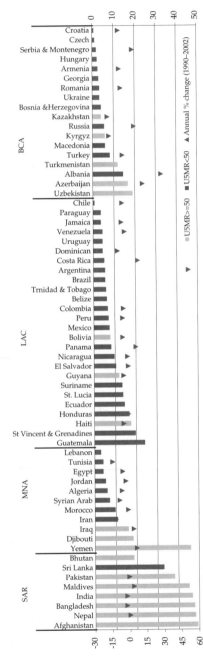

Source: WHO global database on child growth and malnutrition.

Note: U5MR = under age five mortality rate, per 1,000 live births. Prevalence of underweight is from the latest national survey available in each country. The coefficient of a regression that links the natural logarithm and underweight to the year of the survey serves as the average annual percentage change over the period for which data are available. All of the national data available between 1990 and 2002 were used for the estimation. Adjusted prevalence of underweight from national rural data (1990 and 1992) was used for India, as provided by WHO. No underweight data were available for these countries: AFR—Equatorial Guinea; EAP—Marshall Islands, Micronesia, Palau, Tonga; ECA—Belarus, Bulgaria, Estonia, Latvia, Lithuania, Moldova, Poland, the Slovak Republic, Tajikistan; LAC—Dominica, St. Kitts and Nevis; Industrial—Antigua and Barbuda, Republic of Korea, Slovenia.

Although data for the global or regional prevalence of overweight are much less readily available, we looked at data from five countries (figure 2.11) to track when obesity may have started to occur. In Egypt, Zimbabwe, and Peru, where mean overweight rates among children under age five are 12, 7, and 8 percent, respectively, a large proportion of children are already overweight at birth—suggesting again that the damage happens in pregnancy. Weights decline in the first two years of life and then seem to show an upward trend again. Data from Armenia and Uzbekistan are less clear—potentially because of the small sample sizes in the data we reviewed, as evidenced by the very large standard deviations around the means in figure 2.11. These results are consistent with physiological evidence that the origins of obesity start very early in life, often in the womb, though interventions to prevent obesity must likely continue in later life.

Malnutrition is perpetuated across generations. Where undernutrition levels are high, malnourished women or adolescent girls often give birth to babies who are born stunted and small. These children's growth seldom catches up fully in subsequent years. They are more likely to get sick and enter school late, do not learn well, and are less productive as adults. As adults, they are also more likely to suffer from the diet-related diseases such as diabetes, coronary heart disease, and hypertension, formerly thought to be associated only with increasing affluence. Babies born to underweight or stunted women are themselves likely to be underweight or stunted.[25] In this way, undernutrition passes from one generation to another as a grim inheritance.

The key implications for policy are these:

- The best window of opportunity for addressing malnutrition (both undernutrition and, to a large extent, overweight) lies before conception until two years of age (though in the case of overweight, additional interventions are needed in later years). Actions targeted to children older than age two, such as school feeding programs, are likely to have little effect on reversing the damage to brain development, the link with NCDs established in the early years, or on longer-term productivity and human capital formation.
- Access to food is often not the key issue because the food needs of children age 0 to 18 months are relatively small and because undernutrition seems to persist in many households and communities that also suffer from problems of overweight.
- Improving maternal knowledge, feeding, and time for care during pregnancy (to address low birthweight, especially in South Asia) and lactation and improving infant feeding and caring practices, such as exclusive

breastfeeding and adequate and timely complementary feeding, are critical to improving nutrition outcomes. These tasks are closely linked to issues of gender.

All countries with underweight rates greater than 20 percent should get priority for action in nutrition (figure 2.12). Countries with high rates of mortality in children under age five may need somewhat different actions than those with lower rates. Similarly, countries with lower rates of decline (annual percentage change) should be of greater concern, while in those where declines are good, the focus should be on sustaining and scaling up actions.

Notes

1. De Onis and others (2004a); SCN (2004).

2. WHO (2005b).

3. De Onis (2004a); SCN (2004).

4. De Onis and others (2004b).

5. De Onis and others (2004b).

6. Alderman and Behrman (2004).

7. UNICEF and WHO (2004).

8. Kimm (2004); Paneth and Susser (1995).

9. te Veldeand others (2003); Illiadou, Cnattingius, Lichtenstein (2004); Bhargava and others (2004); Zhao and others (2002).

10. Miura and others (2001).

11. Eriksson and others (2001).

12. Ravelli and others (1999); Ravelli, Steing, and Susser (1976).

13. Roseboom and others (2000).

14. IASO (2004).

15. WHO (2002, 2001).

16. IASO (2004).

17. Doak and others (2005).

18. UNICEF and MI (2004b).

19. UNICEF (1990).

20. Pelletier and others (1995); Smith, Alderman, and Aduayom (2005); Haddad and others (1995); Haddad and Smith (1999).

21. Pelletier and others (1995); Smith, Alderman, and Aduayom (2005).

22. Gillespie (2002); Gwatkin and others (2003).

23. Delisle, Chandra-Mouli, and de Benoist (2000).

24. Martorell, Kahn, and Schroeder (1994).

25. Allen and Gillespie (2001).

3
Routes to Better Nutrition

This chapter summarizes what we know about the main interventions for improving nutrition, on both the demand and the supply side, and identifies areas where we need to know more. It outlines two routes to improving nutrition—the long route via birth spacing, food policies, and women's education, and the shorter route via health and nutrition services, micronutrient supplementation, conditional cash transfers, and nutrition education. This chapter also draws two main conclusions about nutrition programs. When it comes to dealing with low birthweight, overweight, and diet-related noncommunicable diseases (NCDs), and with the complex interactions between malnutrition and HIV/AIDS, there are no tried and tested models for effective large-scale programs; action research and learning-by-doing are the priority in these areas. Large-scale HIV initiatives must incorporate attention to nutrition if they are to succeed. By contrast, when it comes to tackling child undernutrition and micronutrient malnutrition, there are several examples of large-scale programs that have led to substantial improvements in nutrition and health behavior and outcomes; scaling up such programs in other countries is the obvious next step. This chapter emphasizes the importance of policy as well as programs. The conclusions are that more attention needs to be paid to the policy process, to ensure that paper policies get translated into action, and that more attention needs to be focused on the unintended effects on nutrition of macroeconomic policies and sectoral policies outside nutrition because they often have haphazard or negative effects that work against the objectives of improving nutrition.

Long and Short Routes to Better Nutrition

A wide variety of policies and programs can improve nutrition (table 3.1). Table 3.1 also illustrates that there are supply- and demand-side approaches to reducing undernutrition. Supply-side approaches include increasing the availability of appropriate foods at affordable prices, improving access to micronutrients, and improving basic health services—immunization, for example, prevents diseases that set back children's growth. There are two types of demand-side approaches. One consists of ways to increase the demand for food, or for health or nutrition services (column 2 of table 3.1). The other consists of changes to behavioral practices related to what is eaten and fed, and to workloads and exercise (column 3 of table 3.1). Most nutrition interventions require changing eating, feeding, or exercise behaviors to have an effect. The fact that many poor children are adequately nourished and many nonpoor children are malnourished emphasizes the critical importance of child-care behavior.

Each country needs to decide on the appropriate balance between the long route and the short route and between supply-side and demand-side approaches to improving nutrition, depending on their capacities, the epidemiology of the problem, and political and institutional considerations. Although both long and short routes are important and should be part of national strategies, this report focuses on the short routes and emphasizes the importance of improving child feeding and caring practices in pregnancy and infancy, for the following reasons:

- Malnutrition's most serious and lasting damage is either during pregnancy or to very young children (chapter 2).
- Several short route interventions can improve child nutrition fast—in two to five years, within the time frame in which politicians need to see results.
- These interventions are affordable at scale by all but the very poorest countries.
- Reducing income poverty or improving the food supply without changing the way young children are cared for often does little to improve nutrition (box 3.1 and see table 1.4).
- Most countries have invested more in food and health than in improving mothers' knowledge and practice of child care and feeding.

Annex 1 lists more than 25 countries where different short route interventions have been successful, while annex 2 discusses long routes to improving nutrition in more detail. The remainder of this chapter discusses some key lessons learned in four types of short route programs—growth pro-

Table 3.1 Routes to better nutrition

Supply-side incentives	Demand-side incentives	Demand-side behavior change
Long routes		
• Primary health services (such as family planning) and infectious disease control • Safe water and sanitation • Policies on marketing breast milk substitutes • Food and agricultural policies to increase supply of safe and healthy food, or of healthier foods • Food industry development and market incentives (disincentives) for developing healthy (unhealthy) food • Fruit and vegetable production • Parks, bike paths, recreation centers	• Economic development (incomes of the poor) • Participatory programs and policy development • Employment creation • Fiscal and food price policies to increase poor peoples' purchasing power for the right kind of foods • Marketing regulation of unhealthy foods	• Improving women's status • Reducing women's workload, especially in pregnancy • Increasing women's education
Short routes		
• Community-based nutrition and health services (community growth promotion programs, community Integrated Management of Childhood Illnesses [C-IMCI]) • Facility-based nutrition and health services (health and nutrition services, and antenatal care) • Micronutrient supplements • Micronutrient fortification • Targeted food aid • Biofortification	• Conditional cash transfers • Microcredit cum nutrition education • Food supplementation • Micronutrient supplements • Food stamps • Targeted food aid	• Maternal nutrition, knowledge, and care-seeking during pregnancy and lactation • Infant and young child feeding • Weight control education • Hygiene education • Promoting healthy life styles (increase physical activity; consume more fruits and vegetables and less salt, sugar, and fat, and so on)

motion programs for young children, low birth-weight prevention programs, micronutrient programs, and food assistance and social protection programs—before summarizing the less well-developed state-of-the-art with regard to tackling undernutrition associated with HIV/AIDS and issues of overweight and obesity.

Community-Based Growth Promotion Programs

These programs' main interventions are nutrition education or counseling (either with or without growth monitoring)—especially concerning maternal care and rest during pregnancy, exclusive breastfeeding and appropriate complementary feeding practices, birth spacing, and how to care for sick children—and links to essential health services. Some programs have also provided micronutrient supplements or food supplements for children and pregnant and lactating women. Throughout this report, we use the term "growth promotion" to refer to such community-based programs.

Box 3.1 Why malnutrition persists in many food-secure households

- Pregnant and nursing women eat too few calories and too little protein, have untreated infections, such as sexually transmitted diseases that lead to low birthweight, or do not get enough rest.
- Mothers have too little time to take care of their young children or themselves during pregnancy.
- Mothers of newborns discard colostrum, the first milk, which strengthens the child's immune system.
- Mothers often feed children under age 6 months foods other than breast milk even though exclusive breastfeeding is the best source of nutrients and the best protection against many infectious and chronic diseases.
- Caregivers start introducing complementary solid foods too late.
- Caregivers feed children under age two years too little food, or foods that are not energy dense.
- Though food is available, because of inappropriate household food allocation women and young children's needs are not met and their diets often do not contain enough of the right micronutrients or protein.
- Caregivers do not know how to feed children during and following diarrhea or fever.
- Caregivers' poor hygiene contaminates food with bacteria or parasites.

Box 3.2 Food security versus nutrition security?

It is important to distinguish between food security and nutrition security, two quite different terms often used interchangeably in the literature. Food security, an important input for improved nutrition outcomes, is concerned with physical and economic access to food of sufficient quality and quantity in a socially and culturally acceptable manner. Nutrition security is an outcome of good health, a healthy environment, and good caring practices in addition to household-level food security. For example, a mother may have reliable access to the components of a healthy diet, but because of poor health or improper care, ignorance, gender, or personal preferences, she may not be able to or may choose not to use the food in a nutritionally sound manner, thereby becoming nutritionally insecure. Nutrition security is achieved for a household when secure access to food is coupled with a sanitary environment, adequate health services, and knowledgeable care to ensure a healthy life for all household members.

A family (or country) may be food secure, yet have many individuals who are nutritionally insecure. Food security is therefore often a necessary but not sufficient condition for nutrition security.

Program experience

Successful, large-scale child growth promotion programs were established as long ago as the 1980s in India's Tamil Nadu state,[1] Indonesia,[2] and Thailand,[3] and continue in Bangladesh,[4] Honduras,[5] Madagascar,[6] and Senegal,[7] among other countries. Such programs lead to a sharp decline in severe malnutrition in the first one to two years, with a slower rate of decline in moderate and mild malnutrition thereafter. A recent cross-country review of successful programs concludes that they led to an average fall in young child malnutrition of one to two percentage points a year—two to four times the 0.5 percent rate calculated as the average trend in the absence of such programs.[8]

Aside from the importance of targeting pregnant women and children under two years of age, those most vulnerable to malnutrition, key lessons about designing growth promotion programs include the following:

- Female community workers are the best people to deliver services because they are less expensive than skilled health workers, on the spot, and able to communicate with mothers better than men. Low levels of formal education are not an impediment to workers' effectiveness so long as they are well trained.

- Because moderate and mild malnutrition are not readily apparent, regular monitoring of children's weights on a growth chart is important, so mothers know whether their children are growing properly and can see the benefits of changes in practices; however, growth monitoring and promotion only work where programs can provide good training and effective supervision in weighing, recording, and counseling mothers, as well as other options for establishing regular contact with mothers.
- Well-designed and consistent nutrition education, aimed at changing specific practices, is key. There are two ways to ensure that recommended child feeding and care practices make sense for poor people in their cultural and economic context (box 3.3).

Breastfeeding promotion and appropriate complementary feeding for children are a central part of growth promotion programs listed as a short route to improving nutrition in table 3.1. But they deserve special mention, both because adequate breastfeeding and complementary feeding could prevent more than twice as many deaths of children under age five as any other intervention[9] and because there are ways to improve these interventions besides growth promotion programs. An important policy intervention is enforcing the International Code on the Marketing of Breast Milk Substitutes, which prevents inappropriate promotion and marketing of commercial infant formula products. A second way to improve breastfeeding is through the Baby-Friendly Hospital Initiative, which applies a 10-step process to improve practices in the labor and delivery wards of hospitals. The tenth step, focusing on follow-up at the community level, has been among the most challenging to implement. A third intervention, peer-to-peer counseling on breastfeeding (such as through La Leche League), has been used throughout the world to extend breastfeeding support to communities.

Where we need to know more

Key questions remain:

- Inadequate training, support, and motivation for community workers are often the main reasons for unsuccessful implementation of growth promotion programs. What would be the most appropriate and sustainable human resource strategies for community health workers to

Box 3.3 Ensuring that new behavioral practices make sense for poor people

Learning from "positive deviants"

A good way to ensure new practices make sense is to see what positive deviants—poor women with well-nourished children—are doing right. Positive practices include everything from breastfeeding from both breasts in Indonesia, to building crude playpens in Bangladesh to keep children from contracting disease from dirty floors, to actively feeding fussy eaters in Mexico and Nicaragua, to adding locally scavenged protein sources to complementary foods in Vietnam.

Source: Marsh and Schroeder (2002); Zeitlin, Ghassemi, and Mansour (1990).

Trials of improved practices (TIPs)

TIPs is a consultative process to develop locally appropriate, culturally acceptable counseling messages that address resistance points and play to motivating factors. Formative researchers visit mothers to discuss child-feeding problems and possible solutions and negotiate changes in practice. They revisit when mothers have tried out the new practices and make modifications depending on what is found to be feasible. Experience with TIPs in more than 15 countries in Africa, Asia, and Latin America shows that trials with as few as 50 families, at a cost of $8,000 to $30,000 per country, can generate valid, programwide findings. For a how-to manual, see Dicken, Griffiths, and Piwoz (1997).

Source: Costing information, personal communication with Marcia Griffiths.

complement health care systems (for example, remuneration and incentives, pre- and in-service training methodologies, and good continuing education for community workers and supervisors) in resource-poor settings where capacity is weak?

- Mothers and caregivers often face challenges in implementing advice on improving the care and feeding of young children. How best can we maximize family and community involvement to help them implement improved child-care and feeding practices at home?
- Food supplementation is expensive, often taking up to 50 percent of the cost of a community-based nutrition program. Supplementing food for pregnant women and adolescent girls, which can improve birthweight and reduce maternal depletion, is especially expensive because they eat

more than children. Under what circumstances is it cost-effective for countries to fund food supplementation for children (or mothers) as part of growth promotion or nutrition education programs, and how best can this food be targeted?

Low-Birthweight Prevention Programs

About 16 percent of infants globally have low birthweight, though these figures vary considerably from region to region.[10] As noted in chapter 2, infants with low birthweights are more likely to die, more likely to become malnourished, and more vulnerable to adult-onset chronic diseases than children born at normal weight. Preventing low birthweight, however, requires attention to more than nutrition. Prematurity, short maternal stature, infections, cigarette smoking, alcohol and drug use, very young maternal age, indoor air pollution, domestic violence, closely spaced pregnancies, hypertension, stress, and malaria all contribute to low birthweight.[11] Some strategies for preventing low birthweight are short route (malaria prophylaxis and treatment programs, iron and folate supplementation, food supplementation); others are longer route (smoking cessation, domestic violence, birth spacing). Some causes are easier to deal with; some can be dealt with through prenatal care; and others require intervention before pregnancy, even as early as childhood.

The technical efficiency of some of the shorter route interventions is relatively well known: iron and folate supplementation, malaria prophylaxis, and food supplementation, when well targeted and implemented, have all been shown to have a positive effect on low birthweight or the health outcomes of the mother-child dyad during and after pregnancy. Other relevant interventions—such as preventing unwanted pregnancy, reaching women before and during pregnancy with appropriate services, overcoming social and cultural barriers to care seeking and behavior change (for instance, women in many regions of the world are thought to "eat down" during pregnancy to avoid having a large baby and a difficult birth), and convincing the woman and her family that her health is worthy of investment—may take longer. Furthermore, because many of the decisions or the circumstances happen either before marriage or soon after marriage, a focus on adolescent girls and newly married couples seems appropriate.

Program experience

Recent evaluation results from the large-scale Bangladesh Integrated Nutrition Project (BINP) project[12] suggest that BINP improved selected knowledge and practices related to pregnancy by 20 to 40 percentage points.

There is some evidence that one of these practices (eating more during pregnancy) is associated with an 88-gram increment in birthweight among those reporting the practice. The evidence suggests little or no additional effect on pregnancy weight gain or birthweight for the population as a whole; however, consistent with theoretical expectations, subgroup analysis suggests sizable effects on birthweight among women who report that they eat more during pregnancy (an additional 88 grams), and an even greater impact among the destitute who report that they eat more during pregnancy (an additional 270 grams).

Such large effects have not been demonstrated in effectiveness trials, primarily because few studies have looked at the mother-child dyad as a combination, instead focusing on the effect on either the mother or the child. Also, most evaluations have looked at a population as a whole, rather than at groups that have a potential to benefit. In the United States, the Women, Infants, and Children Program has successfully reduced low birthweight through a combination of providing food coupons and linking pregnant women to prenatal health care. This approach is akin to the conditional cash (food) transfers referred to in earlier sections, albeit not the same. Its applicability to less developed countries still needs to be tested. Results from the recent community trials of micronutrient supplementation in Nepal also demonstrated that iron and folic acid supplementation can reduce low birthweight by 16 percent, with mixed results on the added value of multiple micronutrient supplementation.[13]

Most mother-child food supplementation programs have documented more success with the child than with the mother. Until recently, the effect of food supplementation on birthweight has been demonstrated primarily in research settings (Narangwal in India, Four Village Study in Guatemala, Dunn Nutrition Centre studies in The Gambia, milk fortification in Chile).[14] The size of this effect was 50 grams of birthweight for every 10,000 additional calories in pregnancy (in Guatemala and Indonesia). Programs have tried creative ways to overcome the cultural resistance to eating more during pregnancy or to resting during pregnancy. The Tamil Nadu Integrated Nutrition Project (TINP) project in India provided a supplementary snack food to pregnant women, which was accepted largely because of its timing, convenience, and image as a snack, though there is little documented evidence of improvements in birthweight in TINP.[15]

Family planning, antismoking, malaria prevention, adolescent health, and reproductive health programs have all had some success, sometimes at large scale, but primarily as vertical efforts.[16] The challenge in preventing low birthweight at large scale is to combine forces, collaborate across departmental lines within and beyond ministries of health, and overcome the formidable problems of health service access, cultural barriers, and women's powerlessness and lack of self-confidence, while combining preventive, therapeutic, and behavioral change approaches. Although this approach has not been demonstrated at scale yet, the potential for success through such integrated programming is there, especially as countries move from projects to programmatic and sectorwide approaches.

Where we need to know more

The evidence for large-scale programs that improve birthweight is much thinner than that for growth promotion or micronutrient programs. Intervention strategies for addressing low birthweight need to be tested at scale in more countries and in more integrated programmatic environments, rather than in vertical project approaches that are rarely sustainable. The scaled-up experience from Bangladesh needs to be reviewed carefully to see how strategies can be fine-tuned to maximize impact. Because food supplementation is a large part of the cost of such programs,[17] the targeting and cost-effectiveness of food supplementation in pregnancy needs to be reviewed very carefully to maximize effects for the mother-child dyad (as opposed to effects on birthweight alone).

Micronutrient Programs

Fortifying foods and providing vitamin and mineral supplements are inexpensive ways to address the widespread problem of micronutrient malnutrition. They can improve economic productivity and economic growth, enhance child and maternal survival, and improve mental development and intelligence in children (chapter 1). "No other technology offers as large an opportunity to improve lives at such low cost and in such a short time."[18]

Program experience

Several countries have successfully iodized their salt supplies, thus reducing goiter and cretinism, preventing mental retardation and subclinical iodine deficiency disorders (IDD), and contributing to improving national productivity. Iodized salt coverage rates of more than 75 percent have been achieved in 26 countries (Burundi, Cameroon, the Central African Republic, Eritrea, Kenya, Nigeria, Rwanda, Uganda, and Zimbabwe; Bolivia, El Salvador, Honduras, Nicaragua, Paraguay, Peru, and Venezuela; Armenia, Kazakhstan, and Turkmenistan; Bhutan, China, Lao PDR, and Vietnam; and Iran, Lebanon, and Syria; see map 1.4).[19] Success with salt iodization, as with other forms of fortification, depends partly on how many manufacturers there are, especially small-scale producers—the smaller the number, the easier it is to develop and regulate the program; how strong the legislative and regulatory system in the country is; and what proportion of the vulnerable have access to commercially fortified foods. Other success factors, more under the control of governments, include the need to:

- Mount public awareness and advocacy campaigns so people know the benefits of using iodized salt.
- Complement the carrot of awareness campaigns with the stick of legislation requiring iodization.
- Back legislation with effective enforcement by ensuring that the amount of iodine in salt is monitored and that only iodized salt is sold in shops and markets.

Developed countries have long fortified milk and breakfast cereals with vitamin A (and other vitamins and minerals), but in developing countries sugar has so far been the most successful vehicle. In Central America, Guatemala's sugar fortification program has virtually eliminated vitamin A deficiency; big reductions have also been seen in El Salvador and Honduras, where fortification was combined with supplementation.[20] Sugar fortification and vitamin A supplementation were also combined in Zambia beginning in 1998, with demonstrated success so far in urban areas.[21] But in much of Africa and Asia the poor do not consume as much sugar as they do in Latin America, so other countries are experimenting with fortifying wheat flour, cooking oil, and MSG (monosodium glutamate) with vitamin A.

Research has shown that vitamin A supplementation can reduce young child mortality in deficient populations by an average of 23 percent.[22] Vitamin A supplements lend themselves to distribution through a campaign approach because children require only two annual doses. Countries as different as Nicaragua,[23] Niger,[24] and Nepal[25] have reached coverage levels of more than 80 percent (see map 1.3). Most campaigns were originally attached to National Immunization Days, but as these are phased out in favor of immunization as a routine part of health services, countries have found other focuses for campaigns—for example, piggybacking on the Day of the African Child and World AIDS Day in Tanzania,[26] or creating twice-yearly National Micronutrient Days, following the example of the Philippines and Niger.

Iron programs to combat anemia have been less successful than iodized salt and vitamin A programs, yet models exist here too. Flour fortification with iron has substantially improved iron status across all population groups in Chile and Venezuela,[27] and rice fortification with iron improved the iron status of school children in the Philippines.[28] A promising large-scale trial of fortifying soy sauce in China also showed that it is a cost-effective way to reduce the prevalence of anemia ($0.0007 per person per year)[29] among all population groups. Several small-scale community-based trials on home fortification with sprinkles for young children in Africa and in Asia have demonstrated that such innovations are feasible and as effective as commonly used ferrous sulphate drops in reducing the prevalence of anemia.[30] The challenge of scaling up these programs remains.

Where anemia is serious and widespread, as in much of South Asia, fortification may not meet the iron needs of vulnerable groups such as pregnant women, and supplementation is also required. Iron supplementation has proved more challenging than vitamin A supplementation because the supplement has to be taken daily and sometimes has perceived side effects. Consequently, there have been problems with the logistics of supply and sometimes with compliance. Indonesia and Thailand have made the most progress in reducing anemia. A practical publication called "What Works in Anemia Control"[31] provides guidelines based on their experience and that of more than 20 other countries that have programs with aspects worth replicating.

Last but not least, the Harvest Plus program is a promising initiative in which the international agricultural and research centers have begun to develop new breeds of staple foods that are rich in key vitamins and minerals using a new approach to fortification termed biofortification (see www.harvestplus.org for details).

Where we need to know more

Key questions remain:

- Under what circumstances is micronutrient supplementation more cost-effective than fortification? How can the two strategies best be combined to complement each other?
- What is the scope for alleviating micronutrient malnutrition through breeding and consuming micronutrient-rich crop varieties and emerging strategies such as biofortification?
- How best can we maximize the opportunities for developing effective multisectoral partnerships (or National Fortification Alliances) with clear financial and operational commitments from all partners?

Food and Social Protection Programs

Program experience

Food assistance and social protection programs can be either long or short routes to improving nutrition. There are lessons about what does and what does not work.

Two types of food assistance seldom work as nutrition interventions. General food subsidies can increase the food consumption of the poor, but they are a prohibitively expensive way to reduce malnutrition (box 3.4). School feeding programs can sometimes be justified in terms of providing an incentive for children to go to school and to perform better, but they are seldom a cost-effective nutrition intervention simply because undernutrition does its principal damage to preschoolers. Yet many governments try to justify school feeding for its nutritional benefits; if this means that school feeding comes out of the health and nutrition budget rather than the education budget, it can have big opportunity costs for programs that improve the nutrition of preschoolers. Nutrition education, iron supplements, and deworming are usually better school nutrition investments than school feeding. Iron supplements and deworming have been shown to improve schooling outcomes as well.[32]

Box 3.4 Food subsidies versus targeted social safety net programs

Countries often resort to general food subsidies as a nutritional safety net program. Unfortunately, these programs are usually expensive and poorly targeted, and sometimes have perverse effects. Subsidies in the Republic of Yemen in the 1990s consumed more than 16 percent of the government budget and almost 5 percent of GDP, and yet only 7 percent of the benefits reached the poorest quintile of the population.[33] In Morocco in the mid 1990s, the wheat flour "subsidy"—really a producer support program—was not only regressive and had a high opportunity cost (the 1.7 percent of GDP it cost could have been invested to generate substantial employment for the poor), but also had a negative environmental effect by encouraging farmers to expand wheat production onto more fragile lands.[34] The good news, at least in the Middle East and North Africa, is that significant policy reforms have since taken place to replace food subsidies with more targeted and effective social safety nets.

By contrast, food subsidies that are regular and significant, but tightly targeted to poor, malnourished populations, can be a cost-effective way to improve household food security—provided they are coupled with counseling services to help ensure that the additional food gets to the most vulnerable household members.[35] Targeting is often best achieved by subsidizing foods that are unattractive to nonpoor people. Furthermore, it has been found that subsidies in the form of food stamps do more to increase food consumption than the equivalent cash transfer. Yet improving household food security is usually a long route to better nutrition, for the reasons given in box 3.1. When can food or cash transfers be short routes to improving nutrition? Experience suggests this happens mainly in three situations:

- *When food assistance is made rapidly available to families who have suffered a serious food security shock, such as a crop failure.* In such circumstances, it can safeguard children's as well as mothers' nutrition.[36] But such aid needs to be well targeted and timely, so success depends on an effective early warning system, easily applicable targeting criteria, and a good storage and distribution network.
- *When food coupons or cash transfers to poor families are made conditional on beneficiaries using health and nutrition services.* Conditional transfers were first tried in Honduras to protect the poor from the shock of structural adjustment, and then adopted by other Latin American countries as human development programs.[37] Evaluations in Mexico,[38] Colombia,[39] and Nicaragua[40] show that conditional transfers, though costly, work when there is political commitment and when they target the right population with the right combination and quality of services (box 3.5). An important lesson is that these programs rapidly increase demand; hence, it is crucial to invest ahead of time in increasing service coverage for the poor, so supply can meet demand. In that context, conditional cash transfer programs can be an important component of both demand-side behavior change and supply-side interventions (see table 3.1).
- *When food supplements for children aged 6 to 24 months are used to educate mothers about the benefits of feeding small, affordable, additional amounts.* As India's experience with food supplementation shows (see technical annex 4.1A), such programs need to be carefully designed if they are to improve home feeding practices and families' self-reliance, rather than becoming welfare entitlements that increase dependence on government.

Conditional cash transfers may be an expensive option for effective nutrition interventions in poorer countries. An argument may be made that where governments may have decided for other reasons to make these transfers, adding a conditional element and linking it to enhanced supply

Box 3.5 Evidence that conditional transfer programs can work

One of the best known programs, Mexico's PROGRESA (now called Oportunidades), aims to break the intergenerational transfer of poverty by encouraging poor families to use education, health, and nutrition services. Between 1997 and 2000, PROGRESA provided cash transfers to nearly 2.6 million rural families (40 percent of the rural total) in return for families participating in services that build human capital, such as schools, immunization services, and health and nutrition education for behavior change. Since 2001, it has also covered 2 million urban families. PROGRESA provides nutrition education, growth monitoring, and micronutrient-fortified foods to children aged 4 to 23 months, malnourished children aged 2 to 4 years, and pregnant and lactating women. Children who benefited from PROGRESA, compared with the control group that benefited one to two years later:

- Had higher median food expenditure and higher intake of energy (7.1 percent).
- Had a better quality diet because they ate more vegetables, fruits, and meat.
- Were about 1 centimeter taller each year.
- Had a more than 10 percent lower incidence of anemia.

PROGRESA's effect was higher among younger children, girls, and children from poorer households. PROGRESA was also seen to have high distributional efficiency among the poorer populations for two reasons: more rural areas were targeted and larger families with more girls got larger transfers.

Source: Gertler (2000); Behrman and Hoddinott (2001); Hoddinott and Skoufias (2003); Handa and Huerta (2004); Rivera and others (2004); Coady (2003).

of services may make supply-side interventions more effective. Yet another variant of conditional cash transfers, a strategy that has not been tried at any large scale, is conditional transfers of food.

Where we need to know more

Most experience with conditional transfers has been in Latin American countries where relatively well-developed service delivery systems mean that supply was able to respond to increased demand. Key questions that remain:

- What scope is there for conditional transfers to work in Africa or Asia, where budgets for transfers are often very limited and health and nutrition services and the capacity to strengthen them are often weak?
- Where governments may have decided for other reasons to make transfers of food or other commodities, such as insecticide-treated bednets, would it be strategic to link these transfers with improved behaviors? Are conditional food transfers an option for improving nutrition?

Malnutrition and HIV/AIDS Programs

In the past several years, an increasing body of evidence has accumulated on the links between malnutrition and HIV/AIDS, and the effect of the two together on economic growth. There is little debate that nutrition plays an integral role in preventing, treating, mitigating, and caring for HIV-positive individuals and affected households and communities (figure 3.1). Yet the strong and devastating interaction between malnutrition and HIV/AIDS—especially in Sub-Saharan Africa, where more than 60 percent of people with HIV/AIDS live and where malnutrition rates are increasing—has only recently been appreciated by policy makers. In a recent consultation on nutrition and HIV/AIDS in Sub-Saharan Africa, WHO and its partners[41] emphasized two points:

- Adequate nutrition cannot cure HIV infection, but is essential to maintain a person's immune system, to sustain healthy levels of physical activity, and to support optimal quality of life.
- Adequate nutrition is also necessary to ensure optimal benefits from the use of antiretroviral treatment, which is essential to prolong the lives of HIV-infected people and prevent transmission of HIV from mother to child.

Two further points:

- Exceptional measures are needed to ensure the health and well-being of all children affected and made vulnerable by HIV/AIDS, with young girls especially at risk.
- Knowledge of HIV status is important to inform choices for reproductive health and child feeding.

Such measures will clearly need to include an increased focus on nutrition.

An issue needing special attention is how to balance the well-known benefits of breastfeeding and the risk of HIV transmission through breastfeeding—a risk that is constant throughout the breastfeeding period.[42] The

Figure 3.1 How malnutrition and HIV/AIDS interact

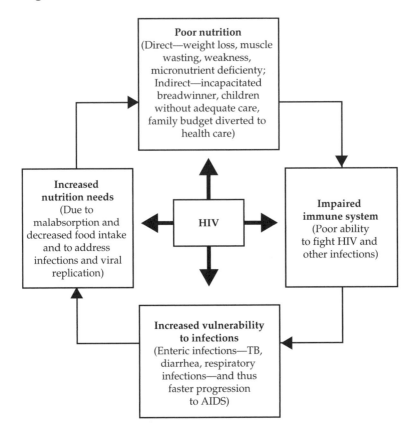

Source: FANTA (2004); modified with information from Gillespie and Kadiyala (2005).

dilemma is that switching to replacement feeding means children miss out on the immunity transmitted through breast milk and so are more susceptible to death or malnutrition from other diseases. The situation is further complicated by the fact that most women in resource-poor settings do not know their HIV status, and there is still uncertainty about the risks associated with different feeding alternatives (such as increased diarrheal disease, stigma associated with not breastfeeding, and spillover effects of formula feeding to mothers who are not HIV-positive). Furthermore, even women who know their status and choose alternative feeding often fall into the trap of mixed feeding (breastfeeding mixed with alternative milks), an option shown to carry the highest risk of transmission. This default to mixed feeding is usually driven by cultural factors, social stigma, or the unavailability of or infeasibility of using breast milk on a continuous daily basis in hot, humid, resource-poor environments. Recent

Box 3.6 Summary findings of scientific review on nutrition and HIV/AIDS

- For uninfected mothers and mothers who do not know their HIV status, exclusive breastfeeding for six months is the ideal practice because of its benefits for improved growth, development, and reduced childhood infections. Safe and appropriate complementary feeding and continued breastfeeding for 24 months and beyond is recommended.
- HIV-infected mothers should avoid breastfeeding when replacement feeding is acceptable, feasible, affordable, sustainable, and safe. However these conditions are not easily met for the majority of mothers in resource-poor settings. If not feasible, early breastfeeding cessation after exclusive breastfeeding (associated with less HIV transmission than mixed feeding) is recommended for HIV-infected mothers and their infants. The age at which to stop breastfeeding depends on the circumstances of mothers and their infants.
- Although there is no evidence to support a need for increased protein intake by people infected by HIV above that required in a balanced diet to satisfy energy need, energy needs do increase by 10 percent in asymptomatic HIV-infected adults and children and by 20 to 30 percent in adults with more advanced disease. For HIV-infected children experiencing weight loss, energy needs increase by 50 to 100 percent.
- WHO's recommendations on vitamin A, zinc, iron, folate, and multiple micronutrient supplements remain the same. Micronutrient supplements are not an alternative to comprehensive HIV treatment, including therapy with antiretroviral agents.
- Viral load, chronic diarrhea, and opportunistic infections impair growth in HIV-infected children, and poor growth is associated with increased risk of mortality. Improved dietary intake is essential to enable children to regain weight lost after opportunistic infection.
- The lifesaving benefits of antiretroviral therapy are clearly recognized. To achieve the full benefits of such treatment, adequate dietary intake is essential. Dietary and nutritional assessment should be an integral part of comprehensive HIV care, both before and during antiretroviral treatment.

Source: WHO (2005c).

findings on the lower risks of transmission through exclusive breastfeed-ing, compared with mixed feeding, warrant the promotion of exclusive breastfeeding until further evidence is available—especially in resource-poor environments.[43]

Program experience

Uganda has led the way in incorporating nutrition considerations into counseling for people living with HIV/AIDS with an excellent set of guide-lines for service providers.[44] A wide range of other nutrition–HIV/AIDS policy options including social protection and rural livelihood interventions are reviewed by Gillespie and Kadiyala (2005), but there is little or no evi-dence about the cost-effectiveness of the options or experience with their implementation at scale. However, there are inherent programmatic effi-ciencies in combining services because the vulnerable groups are similar and a common infrastructure will strengthen coordination, reduce frag-mentation of limited service delivery capacity, and increase the quality of program delivery. RENEWAL (Regional Network on HIV/AIDS, Rural Livelihoods, and Food Security), a recently launched international part-nership, aims to raise awareness, fill knowledge gaps, and help main-stream nutrition considerations into HIV/AIDS policy and HIV/AIDS considerations into nutrition policy (see www.ifpri.org/renewal). The U.S. Agency for International Development (USAID), through its Food and Nutrition Technical Assistance Project (FANTA) and Support for Analysis and Research in Africa (SARA) project, has been instrumental in keeping nutrition issues in the forefront of the development agenda for HIV research. The World Bank is starting an initiative to include nutrition inter-ventions in Multicountry AIDS Projects (MAPs), starting with two coun-tries, Mozambique and Kenya. The objective is to learn from this experience and to scale up to other countries in the region as well as to other non-MAP initiatives, such as President's Emergency Plan for AIDS Relief (PEPFAR).

Although we are still learning how to combine HIV/AIDS and nutrition interventions, neither the virus nor programs to combat it wait for the sci-ence. Large-scale HIV programs are being implemented in many coun-tries, even as research is being carried out and policies developed. The challenges are to speed up research and to incorporate what we know about nutrition and HIV/AIDS as soon as possible into these large-scale programs.

Where we need to know more

Key questions:

- What is the role of improved nutrition in offsetting and mitigating the economic effect of HIV/AIDS in affected households or communities?
- WHO recommends early breastfeeding cessation after exclusive breast-feeding for HIV-positive mothers when alternative feeding is not acceptable, feasible, affordable, sustainable, and safe. What are the effects on growth and nutrition as well as HIV-free survival for children weaned early?
- Under what circumstances is it cost-effective, feasible, acceptable, safe, and affordable to finance replacement feeding for HIV-positive mothers wishing not to breastfeed, and food supplements for people with HIV/AIDS?
- What special nutrition and child care interventions may be needed for the children of parents with HIV/AIDS and single or double HIV/AIDS orphans?
- Daily multivitamin supplements given to HIV-positive adults in the early stage of infection were found, in some studies, to slow HIV disease progression and are therefore suggested to prolong the time before antiretroviral drugs are needed.[45] What is the most effective and efficient regimen for micronutrient supplementation for HIV-positive individuals?
- Could eating more and a better diet, rather than supplements, also delay the onset of AIDS in HIV-positive people and the point at which anti-retroviral drugs are needed? What is the relative cost-effectiveness of nutrition interventions for potential cost savings on antiretroviral drug therapy?
- The target group for HIV/AIDS-related nutrition programs is not just mothers and children—the main clients of other undernutrition programs—but a broader population. What does this mean for the design, management, and cost of nutrition and health services?

Where the prevalence of HIV/AIDS is high, it affects not only individuals and families, but also the development prospects of communities and countries: for example, a labor force reduced by HIV/AIDS may compromise communities' capacity to produce food or to find volunteers for community programs. At the same time, lower productivity means governments have less tax revenue to fund development programs. A corresponding set of research questions at the national and global level includes these:

- When HIV/AIDS reduces financial and managerial capacity at the same time as it increases the need for government intervention, what does this mean for:
  - How governments should allocate investment between short routes to improving the nutrition of those with HIV/AIDS, and long routes such as livelihood creation?
  - How development partners allocate investment between development and social protection programs?
- Most work on the interaction between nutrition and HIV/AIDS has been performed in Sub-Saharan Africa. In Asia, where the next phase of the HIV/AIDS pandemic will be concentrated, how will the interaction differ and how should interventions differ?
- What are the opportunities for scaling up nutrition interventions through large scale AIDS programs/projects such as MAPs and PEPFAR?

Programs to Tackle Overweight and Diet-Related Noncommunicable Diseases

The problems of overweight and diet-related NCDs and ways to tackle them are much less well understood than the interventions for undernutrition and micronutrient malnutrition (see technical annex 3.1 for what is known about the problem and potential solutions). Recent research suggests that obesity in school children and adults often has much earlier roots. Malnourished children are more likely to become obese later in life, and there is a growing body of evidence that suggests that maternal food deprivation or low birthweight may program a child to be more prone to adulthood obesity and NCDs.[46] This—along with changes in eating habits and more sedentary lifestyles—helps explain why many developing countries that had high levels of low birthweight and early undernutrition are now experiencing an epidemic of NCDs.

Program experience

Because obesity is largely the result of changing eating habits, physical activity levels, and life styles, it is in principle largely preventable; and in practice, the high cost of treating obesity-related NCDs means that preventing excessive weight gain or promoting weight loss through a combination of nutrition and health education and food policy actions, which promote a healthier diet and lifestyle changes,[47] are the only feasible way forward. However, if maternal deprivation, low birthweight, and early undernutrition predispose children to later obesity, then incorporating obesity prevention interventions into existing nutrition programs is not entirely incompatible, because undernutrition and micronutrient malnutrition programs mainly focusing on children under age two and pregnant and lactating women will also have a positive effect on obesity. Other important entry points for tackling obesity are ages 4 to 7 years, adolescence, and early adulthood (see technical annex 3.1), so obesity programs inevitably involve a broader target group and hence higher cost and managerial complexity than traditional programs focused on undernutrition.

There is a wide range of potential obesity interventions, ranging from education at the individual level to policy change at the national level (table 3.2). If obesity programs involve health, education, industry, the media, urban planning, transportation, and food and agriculture policy, they will require additional managerial capacity. Yet experience so far is that the seemingly more successful intervention programs, such as Finland's North Karelia project[48] and Brazil's large-scale Agita program,[49] have followed multiple approaches simultaneously. For example, the North Karelia project, launched in the early 1970s to prevent cardiovascular disease through lifestyle and risk factor changes, not only promotes healthy diets (that is, increased consumption of vegetables and fruits and reduced intake of salt), but also generates consumer market pressure for healthier food. Brazil's Agita program targeted school children, older adults, and workers with a combination of special events, informational materials, mass media, training for physical educators and physicians, worksite health promotion, and cooperative ventures with public agencies from several sectors.

One lesson is that health services are not necessarily the main or the best vehicle for achieving behavioral change. Another lesson is that while demand-side interventions (nutrition education) seem the obvious strategy, supply-side interventions such as food policy and pricing of calorie-dense "junk foods" and fruits and vegetables may be equally important. Achieving an appropriate balance between the two may be complicated by conflicts of interest between public health goals (say, eating less energy-dense food) and commercial goals (say, selling more, often energy-dense, products).

A key barrier to scaling up obesity programs is that very few have been well evaluated, partly because different outcome measures have been used and partly because many evaluations focus on changes in clients' awareness, rather than changes in behavior that actually affect obesity. Brazil's program, though better evaluated than most, illustrates this problem; it is clear that the program has led to behavioral change in terms of increased rates of physical activity, but it is not clear what the effects on obesity have been or which components have contributed to the effects.

Table 3.2 The range of interventions for obesity programs

	Intervention types	Where implemented
Communication about diet, exercise, and life style changes	Interpersonal	Local clinic,[50] school,[51] workplace,[52] community[53]
	Mass media[54]	Citywide, regionally, nationally
Policy change[55]	Provide parks, bike paths[56]	Locally
	Promote fruit and vegetable growing and perishable food distribution systems[57]	Nationally
	Lower subsidies on sugar and dairy products[58]	Nationally
	Promote better-quality diet (low fat, low sugar) and market regulation[59]	Nationally

Where we need to know more

- Multitarget, multiagency programs such as Brazil's are relatively expensive as well as institutionally demanding. What is the relative cost-effectiveness of different approaches to controlling obesity and diet-related NCDs in different country circumstances? And, what is the appropriate balance between demand- and supply-side interventions?
- In different country circumstances, how should obesity programs be targeted—on those with existing weight problems, on those at risk of obesity, or on the whole community? When in the life cycle are the best windows of opportunity for targeting programs to prevent obesity and diet-related NCDs?
- There seems a clear link between agriculture and food policies and nutrition and health outcomes. What are the intentional or unintentional effects of policies in other sectors on nutrition?
- Other barriers to progress include lack of awareness among politicians of the seriousness of the obesity problem; lack of awareness among economists and financial planners of its costs; and cultural norms among the obese in some societies that weight is not a concern (there is some

evidence that preference for smaller body sizes rises as countries modernize). In such circumstances, how best can we increase commitment to obesity and diet-related NCD prevention programs, among both policy makers and the public, without crowding out the undernutrition agenda?
- What combinations of integrated interventions can cost-effectively address both undernutrition and overweight in nutrition transition countries? What effective policies that promote healthier foods and diets can also target undernutrition and overweight simultaneously?

The Role of Policy

Nutrition policy—the laws, regulations, and rules that govern public budget allocation and action to improve nutrition—is important, as are programs. For example, an appropriate policy framework is important for the success of programs to reduce obesity (box 3.7). In an ideal world, each country would be committed to a nutrition policy outlining quantitative, time-bound nutrition goals; establishing an overarching strategy; prioritizing specific practical and effective policy reforms and programs; and systematizing progress monitoring and reporting.

The policy process

However, experience with nutrition policy making and implementation has by and large been discouraging. Some countries lack explicit nutrition policies altogether. Others have policies that have not been implemented because they suffer from some or all of the following weaknesses:

- They embrace broad goals without setting specific targets, what interventions will be used to achieve them, and who will be responsible.
- They are not based on analysis of what the different interventions will cost and how they will be financed and implemented.
- They are not linked to investment plans and budgets, or to a monitoring and evaluation process that will inform policy makers on their progress.

Beginning in 2000, the United Nations Children's Fund (UNICEF) and the World Bank jointly reviewed their work in nutrition over the preceding 20 years, with particular emphasis on what they had learned about the policy process.[60] Key conclusions were that policy should be based on a more careful review of country commitment and capacity (both financial and managerial) and that strategies should focus on how they will be implemented[61]—unlike several National Plans of Action for Nutrition developed after the 1992 International Conference on Nutrition, which contained no discussion of implementation. Policies and strategies work only if they are the product of discussion and agreement among stakeholder institutions regarding what they are able and willing to do, and what will be financed and how.

The central importance of the commitment to implement policy can be illustrated by some contrasting country experiences. India developed a national nutrition policy in 1993, a national plan of action for nutrition in 1995, and set up a national nutrition council to oversee implementation. But seven years later the council had not yet met.[62] Thailand paid less attention to formal nutrition policy but based its multisectoral nutrition program on an implementation-oriented investment plan and budget, to which sectoral ministries were committed.[63] Vietnam iodized a substantial proportion of its salt by 1998, even before it formulated policy or legislation for salt iodization—in contrast to the Philippines, which enacted legisla-

---

Box 3.7 The role of public policy

Policy has a potential role in diminishing the poor health and negative economic outcomes associated with the increase in overweight and obesity in developing countries through both demand-side and supply-side interventions.

Demand-side
- Change the relative prices of healthy and unhealthy foods.
- Provide national diet guidelines and food labels to give clearer information about healthy diet and product contents.
- Provide information campaigns to raise awareness of the consequences of poor diet and obesity.
- Develop appropriate multisectoral approaches to address the marketing of unhealthy food to children.

Supply-side
- Increase investment in agriculture to raise productivity and lower the price of fruits and vegetables.
- Eliminate price incentives for high-fat foods and relax quantity restrictions on healthier foods.
- Regulate trade policies to reduce import tariffs on fruits and vegetables.
- Enforce tougher standards on the fat content of processed foods or food consumed away from home.

Source: Excerpt from Haddad (2003); modified with information from WHO (2004).

tion in 1994, but by 1998 had iodized less than 14 percent of its salt. As the UNICEF-Bank review concluded, "policy is what policy does."[64]

Policy choices

Nutrition policy therefore needs to realistically reflect country commitment and capacity and be part of a process to turn policy statements into action. It also needs to address specific policy choices. Thailand was able to mount a successful multisectoral nutrition program because it was strongly committed to nutrition; because it had the necessary management capacity; and because a cultural tradition of community self-help enabled it to expand its national growth promotion program cheaply, using village volunteers.[65] Other countries may not be in this fortunate position: where commitment or financial and managerial capacity are limited, it may make sense to focus in the short run on limited, achievable nutrition goals within one or two sectors. This prioritization will need careful consideration of the trade-offs among the many actions necessary when malnutrition is widespread and holding back development, and the country's capacity to manage these events is limited. Some key priorities, trade-offs, and mismatches are discussed in the next sections.

Short routes versus long routes. One key policy choice is how much to invest in long route investments, as opposed to short route ones. Where finances are tight, short route interventions often offer more bang for the buck. They affect nutrition more directly, and most countries have invested less in micronutrient and growth promotion programs than they have in food and agriculture—despite the evidence from many countries showing that malnutrition exists even in food-surplus areas and among the non-poor (chapter 2). If this is the case, the most cost-effective course of action in the short run may be to concentrate additional funds for nutrition on short route interventions, while complementing these by reallocating existing long route expenditures to have more effect on nutrition. For example, this could be accomplished by:

- Focusing agricultural research and extension on crops grown by women because women's income is more likely to be spent on food-related expenditures for women and children.
- Targeting water and sanitation programs to areas where diarrhea is a major contributor to malnutrition.
- Using nutritional status as a criterion for targeting existing social protection programs.
- Optimizing the availability of certain kinds of foods (fruits and vegetables, sugars and fats and oils, junk foods) and influencing the demand for these foods.

Food supplementation versus health care and micronutrient interventions. There are also important policy choices in striking a balance between short route interventions. Many nutrition programs focus on food supplementation in situations where poor access to health services, poor child-care practices, or micronutrient deficiencies are the main causes of malnutrition. For example, a recent review of nutrition priorities in the Poverty Reduction Strategy Papers (PRSPs) of 40 countries where malnutrition is serious showed that whereas vitamin A deficiency and anemia are public health problems in 35 and 34 countries, respectively, only 13 included activities to address these deficiencies.

Micronutrient programs are an attractive policy choice because of their low cost per head. Where both micronutrient malnutrition and undernutrition are problems, and where countries lack the commitment or the funds to go to scale with multiple short route nutrition programs at once, it can sometimes make sense to scale micronutrient interventions up first, while experimenting with how best to organize growth promotion. Although success with micronutrients is no substitute for investing in large-scale growth promotion programs, it can build the commitment to invest more in growth promotion.

Putting more government money into micronutrient supplementation and budgeting for it within the governments' medium-term expenditure frameworks is particularly important if it is to be sustained: many countries are now dangerously dependent on external grants for these efforts, just as they were dependent on grant finance in the early stages of the universal immunization program. Nevertheless, investment in micronutrient programs must not crowd out attention to general undernutrition, as has been the case over the past decade in some countries. Instead, the capacity and confidence built in the process of implementing micronutrient programs could be used as a building block to implement large-scale community-based nutrition programs that require more complex management skills.

Coverage versus intensity. Experience from programs such as those in Bangladesh, Madagascar, and Mexico shows that the tensions between consolidating the quality of program implementation and the political impetus to expand (or to close down) programs need to be managed very carefully. When political commitment is high, too rushed expansion can compromise program quality. Yet the opportunity and political commitment for expansion does not present too often. Balance is the key.

Some countries have tried to increase the coverage of growth promotion programs—as is often politically expedient—at the expense of quality and the intensity of resource use, whether in the ratio of field workers to clients or the ratio of trainers and supervisors to field workers. This trade-off usually has big costs in terms of quality and effect. A recent review of community growth promotion programs suggests the need for worker-household ratios in the range of 1 to 10 or 20 for part-time volunteers and 1 to 500 for full-time paid workers, and supervisor-worker ratios of about 1 to 20.[66]

Younger children versus older children. Although most undernutrition happens during pregnancy and the first two years of life, and most of this early damage cannot be reversed, many programs.

The poor versus the better off. Though data consistently show that malnutrition is concentrated among the poor, many programs (by design or through faulty implementation) fail to target either the poorest geographic areas, or the poorest people in mixed-income communities. Benefit-incidence analyses should therefore be part of program evaluations and feed into the design of policies and strategies.

Mismatches between the malnutrition problem and the proposed solutions. While most countries do not scale up nutrition programs to any reasonable level (see table 1.8), many do scale up the wrong kinds of programs or interventions. Three mismatches between the need or the cause of malnutrition and the design of programs were identified in India[67] and are common across many other programs:

- *The "food first" mismatch:* Many nutrition programs focus on food security and food supplementation in situations where poor access to health services or poor child-care practices are the main causes of malnutrition.
- *The age-targeting mismatch:* Most undernutrition happens during pregnancy and the first two years of life, and most of this early damage cannot be reversed (chapter 2). Yet many programs continue to expend large resources (especially food) on other age groups (for example, children aged 3 to 6 years, school children). The recent push in Africa for school feeding programs is yet another example of mistargeted resources and is particularly ironic in resource-scarce settings, where it has high opportunity costs.
- *The poverty-targeting mismatch:* Though data consistently show that malnutrition is concentrated among the poor, many programs (whether by design or through faulty implementation) fail to target either the poorest geographic areas or the poorest people in mixed-income communities. Benefit-incidence analyses should be part of all program evaluations.

As mentioned earlier, a recent review of nutrition in the context of PRSPs shows that among 40 countries that have PRSPs, 38 had a micronutrient problem, yet only 23 had specific activities to address micronutrient malnutrition. However, more than 90 percent mentioned food security interventions, even when food security may not have been the major problem.

Intentional and Unintentional Nutrition Policies

Some intentional nutrition policy choices in certain sectors clearly relate to nutrition (box 3.8). In addition, policies in seemingly unrelated sectors can have a strong positive or negative effect on nutrition, in large part through price effects on food and other inputs to good nutrition. For instance, in the mid 1990s, the devaluation of the CFA franc had a large and immediate effect on the Sahelian countries: the urban poor were particularly hard hit, as food prices rose sharply.[68] Another dimension of nutrition policy making is therefore the analysis of the nutrition implications of macroeconomic and sectoral policies, and the development of ways to enhance their positive effects and mitigate their negative ones, for example, by developing compensatory nutrition programs, as Senegal did when the CFA franc was devalued, to cushion the impact on the poor. A wide range of policies can have unintended effects on nutrition (table 3.3).

Box 3.8 Impact of agricultural and food policies on nutrition and health

Agricultural and food policies can affect nutrition and health outcomes both positively and negatively. For example, many Organisation for Economic Co-operation and Development (OECD) countries tend to subsidize grains (such as wheat and maize) more than fruits and vegetables, thereby directly increasing consumption of grains (and indirectly meats), while reducing consumption of fruit and vegetables. A recent review of the European Union (EU) Common Agricultural Policy noted that its support for the cattle sector produced excess dairy products and aided consumption of saturated fats. As a result, diet-related disease, particularly cardiovascular disease, claims more than 7 million years of life annually and obesity-related costs are 7 percent of the EU health care budget.

In Poland, the withdrawal of large consumer subsidies (especially for foods of animal origin) and subsequent substitution of unsaturated for saturated fats and an increased consumption of fresh fruits and vegetables are believed to have decreased the prevalence of ischemic heart disease and mortality from circulatory diseases since 1991.

Source: Gastein Opinion Group (2002); Zilberman (2005); Zatonski, McMichael, and Powles (1998).

Table 3.3 Examples of unintentional nutrition policies

Policy	Potential nutrition effects
Foreign exchange	• Overvalued rates favor urban consumers of imported food at the expense of rural food producers, who are at greater nutritional risk.
Trade	• Protecting local food producers by restricting imports raises consumer prices and net food purchasers (including most poor farmers) are taxed. • Customs and border controls on import of unfortified food where food fortification is mandatory (as with flour in Bolivia and salt in several countries) promotes nutrition.
Environment	• Preserving forests and parks promotes recreational exercise as part of reducing overweight; forests are a major source of foraged food.
Energy	• Taxation or subsidies on domestic fuels affect the type and amount of fuel used for cooking, which affects diet (for example, choosing to cook refined rice instead of sorghum or millet in the urban Sahel).
Employment	• Policies that require firms to offer breaks to lactating women during which they breastfeed their infants.
Roads and public safety	• Safe bike paths and sidewalks in urban areas help promote recreational exercise (as in the "healthy city" program in Bogotá, Colombia).
Agriculture	• Producer subsidies, publicly financed research, and public investments in infrastructure and markets can implicitly subsidize sugar, large animal livestock, oilseeds, and male-controlled cash crops instead of fruits and vegetables, coarse grains, or women-controlled crops, which affect the availability and price of foods and shift household decision-making power away from women. • Regulations or standards of identity of foods, permitted ingredients, purity, safety, nutritional content, labeling, and marketing can promote or inhibit food fortification (as with salt iodization in India), healthy consumer choices (as in Korea), and nutrition knowledge (as in Europe and the United States).
Health	• National health insurance and guaranteed basic health service packages that include (or exclude) growth promotion, micronutrients, and nutrition counseling can affect nutrition (as in Bolivia). • Regulations restricting marketing and distribution of breast milk substitutes, including through hospitals, can encourage breastfeeding.
Education	• Curricula requiring physical education, nutrition, and consumer education (as in Singapore).

continued

Table 3.3 *(continued)*

Policy	Potential nutrition effects
Social welfare	• Social safety nets targeted to the poor ensure access to a minimum diet (income transfers, food stamps, institutional feeding).
	• Efforts to ensure the quality, availability, and affordability of early childhood development and parent education programs that include nutrition.

Program experience

Food policy analysis attempts to systematically analyze the effects of such disparate policies on the food consumption and nutrition of the poor.[69] Macroeconomic and sectoral food policy analysis has been conducted in India,[70] Tunisia,[71] Mozambique,[72] and Indonesia,[73] to name a few, and valuable lessons have been learned about how to effect policy transition in this highly politicized subject.[74] Poverty and Social Impact Analyses (PSIAs) take food policy analysis further, by embedding it in poverty strategies, sectoral reform, and structural adjustment. Within countries, it is important to create the capacity to advise policy makers about the nutrition effects of policies in a focal institution, such as a ministry of finance or a poverty monitoring office.

Where we need to know more

Some basic data gaps make it hard to allocate resources sensibly:

• More than 20 African countries lack adequate nutrition status or trend data.[75]
• Many more countries in all regions lack reliable data on the coverage and quality of existing nutrition projects and programs.

Better cost, affordability, and financing analysis are needed almost everywhere, on several subjects:

• What national interventions cost in different country circumstances.[76]
• What financing can be raised by reallocating expenditures on ineffective programs and which programs can be better redesigned and retargeted.

- What additional public spending will be required, and how it can be financed and incorporated into regular government budgets.
- How benefit-incidence analyses can be made a regular part of program evaluations.

Notes

1. World Bank (1994a).
2. Berg (1987).
3. Tontsirin and Winichagoon (1999).
4. World Bank (2002b); Pelletier, Shekar, and Du (forthcoming).
5. Van Roekel and others (2002); Griffiths and McGuire (2005).
6. World Bank (1999b).
7. World Bank (2001b).
8. Mason and others (forthcoming).
9. Jones and others (2003).
10. ACC/SCN (2000).
11. ACC/SCN (2000).
12. Pelletier, Shekar, and Du (forthcoming).
13. Christian and others (2003); Orsin and others (2005).
14. ACC/SCN (2000).
15. World Bank (1994a).
16. Barros and Robinson (2000).
17. OED (2005c).
18. World Bank (1994b).
19. UNICEF and MI (2004a).
20. Mannar and Shankar (2004).
21. Serlemitsos and Fusco (2001).
22. Beaton and others (1993).
23. Mora and Bonilla (2002).
24. Aguayo and others (2005).
25. Fiedler (2000).
26. Masanja and others (forthcoming).
27. Mannar and Shankar (2004).
28. Mannar and Gallego (2002).
29. Chen and others (2005).
30. Zlotkin and others (2005); Sari and others (2001).
31. Galloway (2003).
32. World Bank (2002c).
33. World Bank (1999a).
34. World Bank (1999a).
35. Alderman (2002).
36. Quisumbing (2003); Yamano, Alderman, and Christiaensen (2005).

37. Coady (2003); Rawlings (2004).

38. Behrman and Hoddinott (2000); Gertler (2000); Hoddinott and Skoufias (2003); Handa and Huerta (2004); Rivera and others (2004).

39. Attanasio and others (2005).

40. Maluccio and Flores (2004).

41. WHO (2005c).

42. Coutsoudis and others (2004); Iliff and others (2005).

43. Coutsoudis and others (1999); Iliff and others (2005); Ross and Labbok (2004).

44. Republic of Uganda (2004).

45. Fawzi and others (2004, 2005).

46. Barker and others (1992); Ravelli and others (1998); Barker and others (2002); Barker (2002); Prentice (2003); Barker (2004).

47. Zatonski, McMichael, and Powles (1998).

48. Puska and others (1998); Puska, Pietinen, and Uusitalo (2002).

49. Matsudo and others (2002); Ramsey and others (2002).

50. NICHM (2003); Sothern and others (2000); Sothern and others (2002).

51. NICHM (2003); Coleman and others (2005); Dowda and others (2005).

52. Coleman and Gonzalez (2001); Doak (2002).

53. Matsudo and others (2002); Kahn and others (2002); Puska and others (1998, 2002); Toh and others (2002); WHO (2000a).

54. Lee, Popkin, and Kim (2002); Doak (2002); Carroll, Craypo, and Samuels (2000).

55. Haddad (2003); Hawkes and others (2005).

56. Neiman and Jacoby (2003).

57. Nugent (2004); Lee, Popkin, and Kim (2002).

58. Nugent (2004).

59. Nugent (2004).

60. Gillespie, McLachlan, and Shrimpton (2003).

61. See especially Pelletier, D., "A Framework for Improved Strategies" in Gillespie, McLachlan, and Shrimpton (2003).

62. Gillespie, McLachlan, and Shrimpton (2003).

63. Heaver and Kachondam (2002).

64. Gillespie, McLachlan, and Shrimpton (2003).

65. Heaver and Kachondam (2002).

66. Mason and others (forthcoming).

67. Gragnolati and others (forthcoming).

68. Diagana and others (1999).

69. Timmer, Falcon, and Pearson (1983).

70. World Bank (2001c).

71. Tuck and Lindert (1996).

72. World Bank (1989).

73. Leith and others (2003).

74. World Bank (1999c).

75. Chhabra and Rokx (2004).

76. For a useful guide to nutrition program cost analysis, see Fiedler (2003).

4
Getting to Scale

This chapter focuses on the challenge of scaling up programs for undernutrition and micronutrient malnutrition in more countries, whether on their own, or as is increasingly the case, as part of health, community development, or other sectoral and cross-sectoral initiatives. There are different options in terms of policy choices, institutional arrangements, and financing approaches, and more analysis on which options are appropriate in which country circumstances will be useful. Several countries have already scaled up successfully, and lessons have emerged from their experiences in managing nutrition programs and organizing services, developing approaches for coordinating with development partners and obtaining financing, and finding ways to strengthen commitment and capacity. The key issue facing the international community is not so much how to scale up or what to scale up, but how to strengthen countries' commitment and capacity to do so.

This chapter reviews lessons from the experience of countries that have tried and succeeded, and tried and failed, to scale up nutrition programs. It focuses on options for managing nutrition programs, organizing services, channeling finance and coordinating financiers, and strengthening commitment and capacity.

Managing Nutrition Programs

The international nutrition community has done less analytical work on these four areas mentioned above than on the efficacy and effectiveness of different nutrition interventions (chapters 1 and 3), reflecting a long-standing bias in nutrition research.[1]

Managing nutrition programs in the field

Of the four areas, there is substantial literature only on how large-scale community growth promotion programs are best designed and managed in the field.[2] Two clear lessons emerge from this literature:

• Involving and, as far as possible, empowering communities are key. This means not only consulting communities about the design of nutrition education and using community workers to deliver services (chapter 3), but also mobilizing communities through well-planned communication programs and giving them a role in designing, monitoring, and managing nutrition services. This was attempted in Senegal's first community nutrition project (technical annex 4.1B).
• Successful programs also pay attention to the detailed micro-level design of management systems for targeting program clients; selecting, training, and supervising staff; and monitoring progress. Monitoring processes that focus communities and implementing agencies on outcomes or results are particularly important. India's Tamil Nadu Integrated Nutrition Project (TINP) (see technical annex 4.1C) and Honduras' Atención Integral a la Ni_ez (AIN) (see technical annex 4.1D) programs are examples of paying special attention to the detailed design of management systems.

Managing nutrition programs at the national level

The many sectors and agencies involved in improving nutrition make management difficult. Because nutrition does not naturally fall under a single line ministry, there has been long-standing debate and experiment (see Levinson 2002[3] for a review) about where its institutional home should be. Experience shows both what does not work (technical annex 4.1E) and what can work. In practice, successful nutrition programs have been managed by a variety of line agencies in different countries, with effective oversight from a variety of coordinating or managing bodies: for example, in Burkina Faso, from a National Food Policy Coordinating Committee; in Madagascar, from the Prime Minister's office; in Senegal, from the President's office; and in Honduras, from a ministerial-level body in charge of coordinating foreign-assisted projects. One set of emerging lessons:

• There should be a clear division of responsibilities among implementing institutions.

- Although oversight agencies should not be given implementation responsibilities, they should be able to influence intersectoral resource allocation so they have a way to give implementing agencies an incentive to
  perform.
- Where the oversight institution is located is less important than that it is
  at a high level and that it is backed by strong political and bureaucratic
  commitment.

Thailand managed its national nutrition program, perhaps the world's
most successful, along these lines as detailed in box 4.1.

Another clear lesson is that, although oversight and control are important, the best results are obtained when stakeholders cooperate as willing
partners, whether in programs involving multiple government agencies,
public-private partnerships such as those for food fortification, or programs
bringing together multiple development partners or cofinanciers. Progress
is being made with technologies for partnership building (see Tennyson
2003 for a recent how-to guide).

Box 4.1 How Thailand managed its
National Nutrition Program

Thailand had no agency in charge of nutrition. The National Nutrition
Program's overall direction was set by a National Nutrition Committee,
chaired by the Deputy Prime Minister, on which the line agencies in the
program were represented. The Committee was served by a small secretariat, headed by the Deputy Secretary-General of the National Economic
and Social Development Board (NESDB, Thailand's planning ministry)
and housed initially in the NESDB and later in the health ministry.
The program was set out in an annual national food and nutrition plan,
allocations to which were controlled by the NESDB, based on line agencies' performance. The Ministries of Health, Interior, Agriculture, and
Education helped draw up their parts of the plan and control its implementation, so they were motivated to perform. The Permanent Secretaries
of the four ministries met once a month to coordinate their work. Thus in
Thailand, it is less appropriate to speak of one multisectoral national
nutrition program than of a set of nutrition programs in different sectors,
run by different agencies.

Source: Heaver and Kachondam (2002).

Where we need to know more

Key areas for further work:

- Best-practice case studies of how countries have organized multisec-toral nutrition program management and partnership building at cen-tral and field levels, and action research on how partnership approaches are best organized and managed in different country circumstances.
- Best-practice case studies of monitoring processes that focus policy makers, implementers, and communities on outcomes and results.

Organizing Services

Because nutrition is not a sector, but contributes to the activities and out-comes in a variety of sectors, nutrition services need to be integrated into existing sectoral programs and build on existing institutional capacity. Using existing capacity is particularly important if nutrition programs are to scale up in Sub-Saharan Africa and other environments where financial and managerial resources are limited.

Fostering public-private partnerships

Countries are increasingly using institutional resources outside government. Food fortification programs harness the institutional capacity of the com-mercial private sector for production and marketing, while the government's role is usually to build awareness, monitor, and regulate. The Micronutrient Initiative (MI), the United Nations Children's Fund (UNICEF), and the World Bank have had successful experience in assisting governments in this area, especially with salt iodization. A new international nongovernmental orga-nization (NGO), the Global Alliance for Improving Nutrition, has been cre-ated to help foster partnerships for food fortification. Similarly, a new Network for Sustained Elimination of Iodine Deficiency is emerging from the Micronutrient Initiative—although questions remain about whether approaches that deal with single nutrients are the best way forward.

Experience from these initiatives is still emerging, and the potential of such public-private partnerships is only beginning to be exploited. In each country, there is a need to identify ways in which the food industry can be involved in designing and supporting implementation of the national nutri-tion strategy. This means developing a multisectoral alliance in each coun-try between industry, the national government, international agencies, expert groups, and other players to work on specific issues relating to technology; food processing and marketing; standards; quality assurance; product certification; social communications and demand creation; and monitoring and evaluation.

As well as working with the commercial private sector, governments are increasingly working through partnerships that use the institutional capacity of NGOs for growth promotion as well as micronutrient pro- grams—as in 1993 in Madagascar, in 1995 in Senegal and Bangladesh, and more recently in Honduras and Uganda. Contracting with NGOs poses a management challenge for governments: NGOs have to be overseen, so developing adequate procurement, performance monitoring, and account- ing capacity in government is essential. But NGOs have proved flexible and many of them, especially locally based ones, are highly motivated and skilled at mobilizing local communities. And because they are employed on a contract basis, they can be phased out once malnutrition rates decline— an exit strategy that is very difficult to implement in programs that rely on government field staff.

Mainstreaming nutrition into sectoral programs and projects

However, most countries lack a strong network of NGOs and need to orga- nize growth promotion services through government agencies. Integrating these services into existing health and child development programs is one logical option. The World Health Organization (WHO) and UNICEF recently commissioned an exhaustive review of more than 700 studies to determine what combination of interventions would have the most impact on child growth and development.[4] Of the 12 interventions this review came up with (see technical annex 4.2A), 5 were in nutrition and 7 in health and hygiene, illustrating why it makes sense to build nutrition interventions into health services (the 12th was in cognitive and social development in early childhood). These 12 interventions now form the core of the Community-Integrated Management of Childhood Illnesses (IMCI) ini- tiative championed by UNICEF and WHO.

Mainstreaming nutrition into health services. Progress is being made in integrating nutrition interventions into health services through several initiatives. One is the WHO and UNICEF–assisted IMCI program, which has made considerable progress in integrating nutrition interventions into health services at hospitals and clinics. The next step, applying IMCI to ser- vices at the community level, is at the pilot stage in several countries. Another initiative is Essential Nutrition Actions, developed by USAID and being implemented by governments and NGOs in several countries. It sets a framework for identifying entry points and tools for integrating essen- tial nutrition actions in policy, health, and community programs. In the Basic Support for Institutionalizing Child Survival (BASICS) projects, nutrition activities are being incorporated into the routine work of health personnel (technical annex 4.2B). Micronutrient supplementation programs have also successfully mainstreamed nutrition through health.

Mainstreaming nutrition into community development programs. But integrating nutrition into health services is not the only option. A complementary opportunity, little exploited so far, is to integrate nutrition into the community-driven development (CDD) programs that are scaling up rapidly in Africa and elsewhere,[5] rather than duplicate institutions for mobilizing and empowering communities in each sector. Integrating nutrition into CDD programs poses risks as well as opportunities,[6] especially the risk that when empowered to choose their own development priorities, communities may opt for investments in infrastructure rather than nutrition. But incorporating nutrition into community development has three potential advantages:

- Growth monitoring data can help communities define their problems and monitor their progress, as in the World Bank–supported Sri Lanka Poverty Alleviation Project.[7] In Thailand, growth monitoring data lead the list of community development indicators that are displayed in every village (technical annex 4.1F).
- Growth monitoring data can help CDD programs target their interventions in different sectors to the families for which they will do most good.
- CDD programs that finance investments in agriculture, income generation, gender, and social protection can help integrate and balance short

---

**Box 4.2 Assessment, analysis, and action:
The "Triple A" process**

The Triple A process was developed in Tanzania's Iringa district and then replicated in several other districts, with assistance from UNICEF. Community workers used child growth monitoring to assess the nutrition situation, identifying families in which there was actual malnutrition and families in which a child's growth was faltering and malnutrition needed to be prevented. They then worked with the family to analyze the possible causes: ill health, poor child-care practices, food insecurity, or some combination. Working with the family and with local government organizations, they drew up a tailor-made plan of action to help the family. Depending on the cause of malnutrition, the intervention might be counseling, referral to the health service, or participation in a livelihood creation, microcredit, or social protection program to improve food security.

Source: UNICEF (1990).

route and long route approaches to improving nutrition at the local level. A practical process for achieving this was developed in the 1980s in Tanzania (box 4.2).

Where we need to know more

- Cultural traditions favoring community service vary, as do the amount of time and energy women have. Where are paid community workers likely to be more effective than volunteers?
- What can be done to build and strengthen the trust of governments to give communities and NGOs more responsibility and accountability for identifying and addressing their development problems, with only selective external help?
- While the potential exists for early childhood development programs to improve nutrition, there has been mixed experience with delivering nutrition services through them.[8] How could such programs be designed to make the most impact on nutrition?

Channeling Finance and Coordinating Financiers

Many countries with serious undernutrition problems need external assistance to help them scale up nutrition services. Whether nutrition actions are sustained and institutionalized depends critically on what vehicles and approaches are chosen for financing them.

Projects

Traditional projects are ideal vehicles for testing delivery strategies before scaling up and have also proved well suited to developing capacity—especially, in the World Bank's experience, when improving nutrition is the primary goal of a substantial project, as in Bank-financed projects in Bangladesh, Honduras, Madagascar, Senegal, and Tamil Nadu.[9] Among their advantages: enough money was spent on nutrition to make an impact; enough technical resources could be put in for effective systems development and learning-by-doing; and managers had a strong incentive to focus on nutrition outcomes because they were the primary project goal. Large-scale projects with an emphasis on capacity building are therefore likely to continue to have a role to play.

But many countries are implementing large numbers of small-scale projects in nutrition, often following different intervention strategies, inadequately evaluated, and overlapping geographically in some areas while leaving big gaps in coverage in others. They leave communities poorly served and governments not knowing which project strategies are most effective. Scarce government management capacity is wasted administering many small-scale efforts and dealing with different donor procurement and reporting requirements. And multiple small-scale projects, flying different donor flags, encourage divided loyalties that make it difficult for government and civil society to build commitment to a national effort to control malnutrition. These major disadvantages suggest that small-scale project approaches are part of the problem rather than part of the solution and should give way to larger-scale approaches and financing.

Sector-wide programmatic approaches

Some countries have made progress toward national nutrition strategies through voluntary coordination efforts. Madagascar, for example, has a voluntary nutrition coordinating group that brings together more than 70 project agencies,[10] reducing project overlaps and harmonizing the nutrition messages sent to communities. Other governments—India is an example—have taken stronger control, enforcing a single community nutrition program model. In the India model, however, the potential programmatic synergies between the reproductive and child health and micronutrient programs (managed by the Health Ministry) and the nutrition program (Integrated Child Development Services Scheme, ICDS, managed by the Social Welfare Ministry) have not been maximized. A third and increasingly widely used option is for traditional projects to give way to program financing, where governments and all development partners cofinance branches of a common national program or vision, rather than small-scale, time-bound projects.

This kind of sectorwide approach (SWAp) is now being adopted in Bangladesh (box 4.3). This should make it easier to sustain and scale up the nutrition program—and to avoid the outcome in Tanzania, where the approach developed by the initially successful Iringa project (see box 0.2) has all but collapsed because the project had no line agency sponsor and its financing was never incorporated into the regular government budget.[11]

Sector-wide programs work best when governments have tested intervention strategies and have developed capacity in procurement, financial management, monitoring, and evaluation—one reason why traditional capacity-building projects still have a place in many countries. Sound monitoring is especially important to the success of sector-wide programs because many of them aim to disburse on the basis of whether output and outcome targets are reached. Linking disbursements to performance creates powerful incentives for managers and workers—but only if the

Box 4.3 Institutionalizing nutrition in Bangladesh: From project to program

Bangladesh's first large-scale nutrition investment was the Bangladesh Integrated Nutrition Project (BINP), a traditional project financed by a $65 million World Bank credit, which expanded a community nutrition intervention piloted by the Bangladesh Rural Advancement Committee (BRAC), a major local NGO. The project focused on improving maternal knowledge and child-care and feeding practices, identified as key causes of undernutrition. The initial investment (1995–2000) was followed up with another investment of $92 million through the National Nutrition Program (2002–6). Financing for scaling up this community nutrition effort has recently been incorporated into Bangladesh's national Health, Nutrition, and Population Sector Program (HNPSP), which will support the government's Health Sector Investment Plan, which includes nutrition (2005–10). The HNPSP is financed by the Government of Bangladesh, with support from 13 development partners, 8 of which (the Canadian International Development Agency [CIDA], the U.K. Department for International Development [DFID], the European Commission [EC], the German Development Bank [KfW], The Netherlands, the Swedish International Development Agency [SIDA], the United Nations Fund for Population Activities [UNFPA], and the World Bank, collectively referred to as the "pooling development partners") will contribute $760 million to a common pool of resources to the government of Bangladesh provided through the World Bank. The SWAp will use common procurement and disbursement procedures and a common monitoring and evaluation system, thereby reducing transaction costs for the government. Other development partners in Bangladesh (including UNICEF, the U.S. Agency for International Development [USAID], WHO, the German Agency for Technical Assistance [GTZ], and the Japanese International Co-operation Agency [JICA], the "non-pooling development partners") will also finance the investment plan, albeit through parallel financing mechanisms. Thus, nutrition will now be financed and managed as part of an enduring government program rather than as a time-bound project. There will be a stronger focus on results: disbursements will be linked to performance, and good performance will be rewarded with extra funds from the pooled financiers. In addition, nutrition is considered key among the six pillars of Bangladesh's Poverty Reduction Strategy Paper (PRSP), thereby further institutionalizing nutrition in the country's development agenda.

Source: Pelletier, Shekar and Du (forthcoming), and World Bank staff.

monitoring system is trusted to reflect reality and if it provides results that feed into the planning and budget process in a timely way.

Programs in multiple sectors

Development financing is also moving away from traditional sectoral projects to multisectoral program financing. More than 50 poor countries have now developed PRSPs, with priorities often financed through multisectoral Poverty Reduction Strategy Credits (PRSCs). A recent review[12] of PRSPs in 40 countries where malnutrition is serious concludes that although most PRSPs mention nutrition issues, they seldom effectively integrate nutrition into strategy. Malnutrition[13] is frequently referred to in definitions of poverty, and nutrition is also often discussed as part of the poverty analyses. Twenty-eight countries used at least one nutrition indicator[14] to measure nonincome poverty; indictors for macronutrient deficiencies such as underweight, stunting, and wasting are most commonly used (even though the technical terms used are not always clear). Six countries also used the United Nations Development Programme's human poverty index, which includes the proportion of underweight children as an indicator of deprivation in a decent standard of living. However, few of these countries follow up with appropriate actions. For example:

- While more than 70 percent of the PRSPs identified malnutrition as a development problem, only 35 percent allocated budget resources for specific nutrition activities. This suggests that nutrition can potentially fit well in multisectoral policy initiatives such as PRSPs; however, because of limited commitment and limited capacity for planning and implementing nutrition actions in countries, it rarely gets funded.
- Many PRSPs identified specific nutrition actions, but they often did not correspond to the type of malnutrition problem. As mentioned in chapter 3, 40 percent of the 38 countries had a micronutrient deficiency problem, but their PRSPs mentioned no activities to address it. By contrast, most countries suggested additional actions to increase food production even when food was not necessarily the limiting factor in improving nutrition in those countries.
- Nutrition actions were rarely prioritized and sequenced on the basis of institutional and financial capacity analysis, or their importance compared with other development needs. Countries with limited development budgets have so far seldom used the PRSP process to face up to the trade-off that doing more in nutrition may mean doing less in other, lower-priority areas.

PRSCs, along with SWAps and CDD programs, are emerging as the dominant approaches to development in smaller, poorer countries, where limited management capacity makes financing development through a smaller number of sectorwide or multisectoral efforts sensible. Integrating nutrition into these vehicles is a challenge now being addressed in countries such as Honduras, Madagascar, and Mauritania, which are scaling up successful nutrition efforts by moving from traditional project to financing through budget support or PRSCs. This experience is too new to have been evaluated; however, an evaluation process must be put in place now, so that lessons can be learned in the near future.

Initial experience suggests that PRSCs may offer a very promising avenue for mainstreaming multisectoral nutrition actions in countries that have already invested substantially in nutrition, and where capacities have been developed through large-scale investment programs. They may be less useful where country commitment to and capacity in nutrition are weak. The dilemma is that while such countries do not have the capacity to implement large numbers of individual projects and need to explore multisectoral alternatives, making nutrition a small part of a multisectoral program may be tantamount to sidelining it. In such cases, where commitment and capacity for nutrition are weak and yet it may have been included in the PRSPs/PRSCs, several options need to be systematically explored and documented:

- A phased approach, beginning with a standard investment project or projects in nutrition to build capacity, followed by mainstreaming in a PRSC.
- Ensuring that nutrition activities get appropriate attention in PRSCs by giving them clear objectives and progress indicators, and by incorporating processes for progress monitoring by a variety of stakeholders—politicians, government departments, program clients, and the media.
- Complementing a nutrition component of such a PRSC with an additional technical assistance project for nutrition capacity building.

Where we need to know more

More work is needed to document country experience with:

- How to integrate nutrition better into health and other sectoral programs and into PRSPs, PRSCs, SWAps, and other new financing and coordinating approaches, while paying adequate attention to the details of behavioral change communication, management, and accountability that are critical for the success of nutrition activities.
- How best to test and evaluate new strategies and develop management capacity in countries where development financing has moved from a project to a program approach.

Box 4.4 Five steps toward integrating nutrition in country PRSPs

Step 1: Determine whether the country has a nutrition problem of public health significance (see annex 1 or technical annex 5.6 for a list of countries):

- If yes, a strong rationale for including nutrition issues in the PRSP exists.
- If yes, develop a case for prioritizing nutrition over other sectors in the country PRSP.
- If not, prioritize other sectors and see if and how nutrition issues fit.

Step 2: If nutrition issues are important:

- Review the size and nature of the nutrition problem (see annex 1 for basic information).
- Using levels of malnutrition estimated in annex 1, calculate estimated productivity losses attributable to malnutrition (both undernutrition and overweight), and analyze cost-benefit of addressing malnutrition.[a]

Step 3: Identify the (possible) causes of malnutrition:

- This information may be available in country.
- If not, commission some analytical work—Demographic Household Survey data are usually a good source for these analyses; also check for other data sets such as Multiple Indicator Cluster Surveys and Living Standards Measurement Surveys.[a]

Step 4: Set up working groups to:

- Identify appropriate objectives for nutrition in the country.[a]
- Select strategies and actions that will respond to the size and nature of the nutrition problem.[a]
- Prioritize proposed actions so they match the epidemiology of the problem and the country capacity.
- Lay out appropriate institutional arrangements for supporting the implementation of nutrition activities across sectors.[a]
- Identify monitoring and evaluation arrangements and capacity development plans.[a]

Step 5: Allocate reasonable funds and resource them through subsequent PRSCs:

- Support implementation.
- Strengthen capacity and implementation through a learning-by-doing approach.

Source: Excerpts from Shekar and Lee (2005).
a. These steps can be built into the PRSP/PRSC implementation process; however, consider laying out these steps in the PRSP.

- A related question (addressed in chapter 3) is to explore the opportunities for scaling up nutrition actions/interventions through Multicountry AIDS Projects (MAPs) and other large-scale AIDS initiatives such as the President's Emergency Plan for AIDS Relief (PEPFAR).

Strengthening Commitment and Capacity

If short route nutrition interventions have high benefit-cost ratios and many of them are quite affordable (chapter 1), why have most countries failed to scale them up—and why have most development assistance agencies put few resources into them? The key constraints appear to be weak commitment and capacity. Of the two, commitment is the binding constraint, since the precondition for developing capacity is commitment to do so.

Strengthening commitment

Country commitment to combating malnutrition can be weak for a variety of reasons (box 4.5). A recent report[15] suggests ways to assess commitment and reviews how some countries with successful nutrition programs built the commitment to scale up. One or a few champions of nutrition—people with the ear of policy makers and capable of carrying out evidence-based advocacy—built partnerships of individuals and institutions that can influence politicians and implementing agencies to press for increased budgets for nutrition programs. They did this by convincing others that improving nutrition was essential to achieving their own goals—whether political stability, national security, developing education, industry or agriculture, or international competitiveness.

Effective communication is the key to building commitment. In Bangladesh, a PROFILES analysis (Academy for Educational Development [AED] process for nutrition advocacy, box 4.6) helped convince financial decision makers of the importance of investing in nutrition. A film from a pilot project, showing children suffering from malnutrition and how village women could run an effective growth promotion program for them, helped bring key politicians on board. In Uganda, politicians promoted the Early Childhood Development and Nutrition project through a specially created Parliamentary Advocacy Committee, and were given on-camera training in how to communicate to the media about the project.[16] These experiences show how important it is to use different communication strategies to win the support of different stakeholders.

But there is more to strengthening commitment than good communication, as shown by Thailand's experience developing its community nutrition program (technical annex 4.1G), and China's developing its salt fortification program (technical annex 4.1H). Also important in varying

---

**Box 4.5 Ten reasons for weak commitment
to nutrition programs**

- Malnutrition is usually invisible to malnourished families and
  communities.
- Families and governments do not recognize the human and economic
  costs of malnutrition.
- Governments may not know there are faster interventions for combat-
  ing malnutrition than economic growth and poverty reduction or that
  nutrition programs are affordable.
- Because there are multiple organizational stakeholders in nutrition, it
  can fall between the cracks.
- There is not always a consensus about how to intervene against
  malnutrition.
- Adequate nutrition is seldom treated as a human right.
- The malnourished have little voice.
- Some politicians and managers do not care whether programs are
  well implemented.
- Governments sometimes claim they are investing in improving
  nutrition when the programs they are financing have little effect on
  it (for example, school feeding).
- A vicious circle: lack of commitment to nutrition leads to underinvestment in nutrition, which leads to weak impact, which reinforces lack
  of commitment since governments believe nutrition programs do
  not work.

Source: Abridged from Heaver (2005b).

---

degrees in different country circumstances are building informal con-
stituencies in the civil service and in civil society, as well as with industry
where appropriate; management arrangements that provide incentives for
implementers; appropriate choices of financing vehicles; effective performance monitoring; policy environments conducive to reform; strong legislative and regulatory frameworks; and support from external development
partners working together. Efforts to organize civil society in support of
nutrition are particularly critical. Thailand's success in mobilizing civil
society helps explain how it sustained commitment to its nutrition program for more than 25 years. By contrast, in Bangladesh, Tamil Nadu, and
Tanzania, there has been little public pressure to keep initially successful programs on track when government or development partner commitment
has faltered.

Box 4.6 PROFILES

PROFILES is a computer-based program for calculating the benefits from improving nutrition in terms of mortality and disease reduction, increased productivity and wages gained, and reductions in spending on social sector programs. Financial decision makers particularly appreciate the program's simulation facility, which allows them to instantly see the implications for the economy of different levels of achievement in improving nutrition.

PROFILES estimates the far-reaching consequences of malnutrition, assessing the short- and long-range benefits of combating nutritional deficiencies, and helps in communicating these findings to decision makers. Over the past 10 years, PROFILES has been used in 25 countries (Bangladesh, Ethiopia, Ghana, Guatemala, India, Russia, and Gaza, to name a few) and a recent evaluation of PROFILES shows that it is an effective tool for:

*   Raising awareness about nutrition, promoting coalitions in support of nutrition, and building consensus that nutrition is a priority.
*   Building capacity and developing the leadership skills of nutrition advocates.
*   Promoting more comprehensive nutrition strategies, leveraging new resources for nutrition, and better targeting existing resources.

In Ghana, for example, a team of nutrition and health professionals from various government ministries, universities, and NGOs used PROFILES to estimate that 5,500 infants were dying per year as a result of suboptimal breastfeeding practices. The use of PROFILES with other initiatives helped nutrition advocates address poor infant feeding practices and helped mobilize the government to include breastfeeding and nutrition programs among its top five child survival priorities, as well as make it the top priority of the Ghana Vision 2020 health sector strategy. For further details, see www.aedprofiles.org.

Source: Excerpt from AED (2003).

Strengthening capacity

The literature on strengthening management and implementation capacity in nutrition is limited.[17] This section develops just two themes among many needing attention in this field—the usefulness of distinguishing between capacities that can be built during implementation and capacities that need to be developed before scaling up, and the need to pay greater attention to issues of governance as part of capacity building.

When and how to build capacity. Most countries that develop success-ful nutrition programs do not wait to build capacity before scaling up. After short pilot activities to develop effective strategies (a year in the case of Tamil Nadu and Bangladesh), they expand rapidly. Thailand mobilized half a million volunteers in just a few years. The nutrition champions knew they needed to move fast to take advantage of political commitment—a need that must be balanced against the risks of too rapid expansion, which can jeopardize funding and commitment if the program fails to deliver results.

With this trade-off in mind, Matta, Ashkenas, and Rischard (2000) are developing an approach called "building capacity through results," in which systematic capacity building is built into the implementation process. Program implementation is broken down into steps; an analysis is made of what capacities, and whose, need to be developed to achieve the next step; and capacity development activities are limited to only those needed to achieve the next step. This approach means that capacity development automatically responds to operational needs, and managers have an incen-tive to focus on it because each capacity-building activity produces an immediate, tangible, improved outcome—unlike traditional institutional development activities, which are often disconnected from operations and given low priority.[18]

This approach can be systematically used to build capacities in com-munity mobilization, field-level training, and supervision during program implementation. However, a small number of key capacities are needed before programs expand. In addition to strengthening procurement and financial management capacity (now usually routinely included), up-front attention is required to the capacities for:

- Communicating effectively, which is critical for strengthening the com-mitment of development partners, governments, and civil societies to nutrition, in turn a precondition for increasing investment.
- Analyzing the relative cost-effectiveness of nutrition programs and ser-vice delivery approaches, key to ensuring the right investment decisions are made.
- Carrying out quality baseline studies, so countries can evaluate down the line how well their investment has paid off.

The need for more attention to issues of governance and corruption. A review of institutional development interventions in a sample of World Bank–assisted health and nutrition projects in Africa[19] found that their focus was mainly on three or four of ten possible types of intervention: adding staff and physical and financial inputs; providing training and tech-nical assistance; introducing new technologies; and changing coordination mechanisms. The shortage of trained human resources, especially in

Sub-Saharan Africa, means that traditional, training-oriented, capacity development interventions will remain important. But equally salient in both Africa and South Asia, where malnutrition is concentrated, are problems of weak governance and corruption.[120]

To address these issues, governments and development partners may need to focus more on six capacity development interventions that this study found to be less widely implemented:

- Increasing particular stakeholders' voice in planning and implementation.
- Altering the balance between public and private sectors in service delivery.
- Reforming specific organizational systems.
- Changing or enforcing laws, rules, or regulations.
- Changing attitudes, values, organizational cultures, or incentives and disincentives.
- Providing information and increasing accountability.

Recent work on education in Africa points to high returns from improvements in the governance of social services in countries where corruption is institutionalized.[21]

Where we need to know more

The priority needs are for:

- Practical methodologies for assessing and strengthening commitment and institutional capacity.
- Case studies of successful attempts to assess and strengthen commitment and capacity, and to deal with problems of poor governance and corruption.

Notes

1. Berg (1992).

2. Jennings and others (1991); Gillespie, Mason, and Martorell (1996); ACC/SCN (1997); Jonsson (1997); Hunt and Quibria (1999); Tontsirin and Gillespie (1999); Allen and Gillespie (2001); Heaver (2002).

3. A summary of this paper can be found in Gillespie, McLachlan, and Shrimpton (2003).

4. Hill, Kirkwood, and Edmond (2004).

5. Gillespie (2004).

6. Heaver (2003b).

7. World Bank (1998); Ranatunga (2000).

8. Heaver (2005a).

9. Heaver (2005a).

10. Rokx (2000).

11. Dolan and Levinson (2000); a summary of this paper can be found in Gillespie, McLachlan, and Shrimpton (2003).

12. Shekar and Lee (2005).

13. Not only the explicit term "malnutrition" and its indicators stunting and underweight, but also implicit terms such as "food insecurity," "insufficient food," and "hunger" are used in definitions of poverty.

14. One of the most commonly used income poverty indicators, percentage of food-poor is the proportion of households whose annual per capita expenditure is not enough to buy a basket of food products that ensures the minimum energy requirement.

15. Heaver (2005b).

16. Elmendorf and others (2005).

17. For a tentative conceptual framework for assessing and strengthening capacity in nutrition, see Gillespie (2001); for a discussion of issues in nutrition management and capacity development, see Heaver (2002).

18. Johnston and Stout (1999).

19. Orbach and Nkojo (1999).

20. For example, at different times and in different places, World Bank–supported nutrition programs have suffered from attempts by program managers to use political influence to hire NGOs and community workers who do not meet program recruitment criteria; demand kickbacks for contracts, for recruitment, or for promptly processing expenditure claims; fix the bid prices of supplementary food and medicines; and supply low-quality weighing scales or food, permitting contractors to finance kickbacks from the excess profits.

21. Reinikka and Svensson (2004).

5
Accelerating Progress in Nutrition: Next Steps

Chapter 1 outlined why we must invest in nutrition. Chapter 2 detailed the enormous size and the extensive scope of the nutrition problem (both underweight and overweight) at global, regional, and country levels to further strengthen the case for investing in nutrition. Chapter 3 outlined how best to tackle malnutrition. Chapter 4 focused on the challenge of scaling up programs for undernutrition and for micronutrient malnutrition in more countries, incorporating nutrition in rapidly expanding HIV/AIDS initiatives, while starting to address issues of overweight and diet-related noncommunicable diseases (NCDs), where relevant.

This chapter proposes that to accelerate progress in nutrition, development partners, in collaboration with developing countries, need to convene around a common agenda in nutrition and agree to support this agenda through a coordinated, focused set of actions in two areas:

- *Scaling up action in countries by addressing the three key operational challenges: mainstreaming nutrition in country strategies and approaches; reorienting existing large-scale programs to maximize their effects; and building global and national commitment and capacity for enhancing investments in nutrition.*
- *Supporting a coordinated set of priorities for action research and learning-by-doing in mainstreaming nutrition in the development agenda, strengthening and fine-tuning delivery mechanisms, and strengthening the evidence base for investing in nutrition.*

Without this kind of coordinated and focused action by development partners and developing countries, no significant progress in nutrition can be expected and the Millennium Development Goals (MDGs) will continue to be compromised in the countries and among the people who need them the most.

Uniting Development Partners around a Common Nutrition Agenda

Development partners supporting nutrition

The principal development partners that support nutrition at the global or national levels are shown in figure 5.1. Most development partners supporting nutrition focus on food security, agriculture, and rural development, followed by HIV/AIDS and nutrition as part of maternal and child health services (technical annexes 5.1 and 5.2 outline partners' primary focus areas). Addressing micronutrient deficiencies, seizing the window of opportunity to address undernutrition among young children, and controlling overweight and obesity come lower in the current priorities of most partners. Few agencies are working toward mainstreaming nutrition into Poverty Reduction Strategy Credits (PRSCs), Poverty Reduction Strategy Papers (PRSPs), or sectorwide approaches (SWAps), or even across other intersectoral programs such as gender and community-driven development (CDD) programs.

Figure 5.1 Principal development partners supporting nutrition

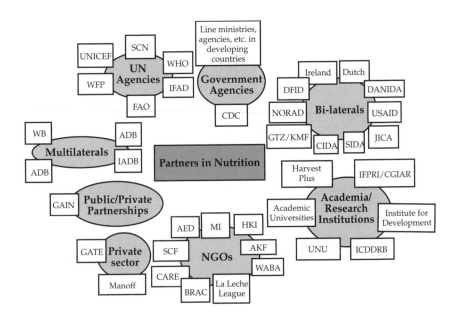

Most partners support capacity development activities in some form, but much of this effort goes into training nutritionists to be better nutritionists, rather than in orienting key government planning, finance, and economics staff toward nutrition and building commitment and support for nutrition in ministries of finance and planning. Though some agencies are actively building commitment, their efforts are mainly limited to narrow focus areas (such as breastfeeding for the World Alliance for Breastfeeding Action and La Leche League, and micronutrient fortification in selected countries for the Global Alliance for Improving Nutrition [GAIN]). The continuing low level of global interest in general nutrition is evidence that commitment building has been neglected; the fact that many of the agencies reviewed in technical annexes 5.1 and 5.2 have no specific nutrition policies or focus makes it even more evident that nutrition has been marginalized in the development agenda, even by development partners.

Each country needs to drive its own investment agenda and hence should lead the repositioning of nutrition in the development agenda that is proposed in this report. When countries request help in nutrition, the role of development partners is to respond, first by helping countries develop a shared vision and consensus on what needs to be done, how, and by whom, and then by providing financial and other assistance. Nevertheless, in chapter 4 we argued that much of the failure to scale up action in nutrition results from a lack of sustained government commitment to action and hence low demand for assistance in nutrition. In this situation, the role of the development partners must extend beyond responding when requested to do so by governments, to using their combined resources for analysis, advocacy, and capacity building to encourage and influence governments to put nutrition higher on the agenda wherever it is holding back achievement of the MDGs, poverty reduction, and human capital formation. This role can be fulfilled only if the development partners share a common view of the malnutrition problem and broad strategies to address it and speak with a common voice (box 5.1).

Building a shared vision and consensus on actions does not imply that there should be no discussion or dissenting voices or new research. Instead, we propose that the approach to cooperation and consensus should differ in the political and programmatic realms. In the political realm, key development partners must forge a consensus on the "big picture" issues that drive and sustain political commitment to investing in nutrition at global and national levels. In the programming realm, partners must institute a culture of inquiry that derives from action research, monitoring, and evaluation—and that drives stakeholders at all levels to continuously reorient and fine-tune programs and investment strategies to maximize impact, within the framework of a broad strategic consensus.[1] Although previous efforts at uniting development partners have not always been successful, we hope that this distinction between the political and the programmatic realms will help lay the groundwork for successful consensus building as nutrition is repositioned at the center of the development agenda.

Box 5.1 Lessons for nutrition from HIV/AIDS

Some lack of focused interest and support for nutrition may derive from the disadvantages inherent in multisectoral problems and solutions, but successful examples from HIV/AIDS may offer lessons for scaling up nutrition efforts. The Multicountry HIV/AIDS Program (MAP) was jump-started by the World Bank committing $1 billion in little more than three years and creating an enabling environment for major inputs from other partners. This happened because Bank leaders spoke out forcefully and regularly so the issue became a "must" on national agendas, and dedicated Bank funds and staff provided consistent support, and a mechanism supported by the Bank coordinated the relevant partners (primarily UN agencies through the Joint United Nations Programme on HIV/AIDS [UNAIDS]). Such a potential mechanism exists for nutrition through the United Nations' Standing Committee on Nutrition (SCN)—but for the SCN to play a coordination role would require major changes in its mandate. Other more operational mechanisms may need to be explored.

Further lessons are embodied in the MAP interim review undertaken in 2004. It identified eight critical MAP elements that provide a simple framework—one that could apply to future efforts in nutrition:

- Government commitment and governance, particularly the role of national leadership (in nutrition this is embodied in resolving institutional and commitment-building issues).
- National HIV/AIDS strategies and frameworks linked to resource allocation (National Plans of Action for Nutrition have been largely theoretical, unlinked to national resources, and divorced from assessments of national capacities).
- The multisectoral approach, including but not limited to the health sector.
- Community engagement (may need to be considered in a review of human resources for nutrition at community levels, among other issues).
- Strengthened monitoring and evaluation.
- Donor collaboration and coordination.
- Bank instruments—and the links from MAP projects to programmatic loans and health sector investments.
- Implementation experience.

Three Key Operational Challenges to Scaling Up

To more effectively address the malnutrition challenge, actions must be scaled up. To do so, three key operational issues must be addressed. They are to mainstream nutrition interventions into programs (rather than projects) in health, agriculture, and other sectors; to reorient some existing large-scale nutrition investments that are not achieving the desired effect; and to build the commitment and capacity required to underpin the scaling-up and reorientation needed. Some tools to help development partners decide on priorities for scaled-up action follow this discussion.

Mainstreaming nutrition in country strategies and program approaches

As outlined in chapter 4, a new programming environment is emerging globally and nationally. The move from projects to programs, from financing and implementing vertical disease-specific projects to SWAps and budget support, as well as a reinvigorated focus on multisectoral action, poverty reduction, and equity issues, are all part of this new environment. The roles of civil society and the private sector are becoming more important. The focus on results has never been higher on the agenda of both development partners and developing countries. These changes call for new approaches in taking the nutrition agenda forward, especially in the following areas.

Repositioning nutrition appropriately in country development strategies. Countries need to recognize that nutrition is not a consumption issue; nor is it primarily a question of welfare. Strategic nutrition investments can contribute to human capital formation and can thereby drive economic growth. Nutrition is an integral part of the first MDG, which aims to reduce poverty and hunger. While many countries are on track in reducing income poverty, most are not on track in improving nonincome poverty (malnutrition and hunger). Without direct investments in nutrition, they will continue to be off track not only on the first MDG, but also on the health, HIV/AIDS, education, and gender MDGs (chapters 1 and 2). This critical recognition is the most important issue in repositioning nutrition in country development strategies and within the agendas of development partners.

Many evaluations have rightfully cautioned that intervention strategies must be context-specific,[2] so we do not subscribe to a prescriptive approach. Each country's strategy and actions for improving nutrition will look different. In particular, each country needs to find a balance of interventions in food, health, and caring practices that is appropriate to its situation—in terms of the type and seriousness of malnutrition, where past nutrition investments have gone, and the country's commitment and capacity to act. (See figure 5.2 for a practical tool for helping countries make policy choices for investing in nutrition, and box 5.2 for some specific suggestions about priorities when commitment or capacity are weak.) We do not propose a global "one size fits all" approach to addressing malnutrition; however, we do recommend that when developing national or regional strategies, countries and their development partners pay special attention to the following efforts:

- Focusing strategies and actions on the poor to address the nonincome aspects of poverty reduction that are closely linked to human development and human capital formation.
- Focusing interventions on the window of opportunity—conception through the first two years of life—because this is when irreparable damage occurs.
- Improving mother- and child-caring practices to reduce the incidence of low birthweight, and to improve infant-feeding practices, including exclusive breastfeeding and appropriate and timely complementary feeding, because many countries and development partners have neglected to invest in such programs.
- Scaling up micronutrient programs because of their widespread prevalence, effect on productivity, affordability, and extraordinarily high benefit-cost ratios.
- Building on the country capacities developed through micronutrient programming to extend actions to community-based nutrition programs.
- Working to improve nutrition not only through health, but also through appropriate actions in agriculture, rural development, water supply and sanitation, gender, social protection, education, and CDD.[3]
- Strengthening investments in the short routes to improving nutrition, yet maintaining a balance between the short and the long routes.
- Integrating appropriately designed and balanced nutrition actions in country assistance strategies, SWAps in multiple sectors, MAPs, and PRSPs.

Development partners can assist by:

- Helping countries identify appropriate institutional arrangements for policy development, cost-effectiveness and affordability analysis, and investment planning.
- Providing technical assistance and capacity-building support in these areas if needed.

Accelerating the move from project to more coordinated program approaches. Multisectoral PRSPs, PRSCs, and SWAps offer an opportunity to mainstream and scale up nutrition. Development partners can help countries take advantage of this opportunity by moving from financing

Box 5.2 What to do when

Financial capacity is weak:

- Vitamin and mineral supplementation (vitamin A, iodine, iron).
- Food fortification.
- Immunization.
- Oral rehydration therapy.
- Deworming.
- Community-Integration Management of Childhood Illnesses (IMCI), including nutrition.
- Growth promotion, if it can be added to an existing outreach system.

Managerial capacity is weak:

- Immunization and oral rehydration therapy.
- Vitamin A supplementation as an add-on to immunization.
- Food fortification (provided there is a manageable number of food manufacturers).
- Growth promotion, if it can be added to an existing outreach system.
- Leverage scarce government capacity by:
  - Contracting services out to NGOs, if available
  - Using community organizations to deliver services.

Commitment is weak:

- Reduce risk by choosing just one or two interventions in one or two government departments where champions can be found.
- Start with interventions that are relatively cheap and easy to manage, such as vitamin A and iodine supplementation.
- Pilot interventions in a small area, where speedy, commitment-boosting results can be assured without government spending too much money.
- Invest in analysis and evidence-based advocacy to strengthen country commitment rather than in donor-driven projects that will not be sustained without country ownership.

Source: Excerpt from technical annex 5.4.

small-scale, donor-driven projects to partnering in large-scale, country-driven programs; by agreeing on how each agency can best support developing country governments in terms of its comparative advantage in financing, technical expertise, or presence; and by reducing the government's aid management burden through common procurement, accounting, and reporting procedures. This is beginning to happen in some countries, showing that it can be done:

- In Bangladesh through the recently approved Health, Nutrition, and Population Sector Program (HNPSP), 13 donors have agreed to pool their funds for a SWAp—of which a substantial proportion will go to nutrition. Nutrition is also a key element of the draft PRSP in Bangladesh. All this builds on experience gained through previous traditional projects—the Bangladesh Integrated Nutrition Project (BINP) and the National Nutrition Project.
- In Madagascar, nutrition is being mainstreamed and scaled up through the PRSC, building on experience from the SEECALINE project.
- In Ethiopia, the government is developing a national nutrition strategy with coordinated support from several partners (The United Nations Children's Fund [UNICEF], the Canadian International Development Agency [CIDA], the U.S. Agency for International Development [USAID], the International Food Policy Research Institute, the World Bank, and others). The strategy, which was a condition to be met before the next PRSC, can provide a focus for coordinated donor support in the country and could be resourced from the next PRSC as well as from coordinated donor resources for different elements.

Reorienting existing large-scale investments to maximize impact

While most countries have failed to mount large-scale programs to improve nutrition, some have made substantial investments whose effects are less than they could be. This usually happens because the quality of implementation is poor, or because there is a mismatch between the causes of malnutrition and the priorities of the programs to address it, as outlined in chapter 4. In many cases, even where the need to change design and strategy is recognized, bureaucratic and political resistance to change often makes programs more inflexible than they need to be.

Improving implementation quality. Poor implementation quality can have a variety of causes: implementation capacity in general may be weak; some specific aspects of program management such as worker training may be weak; or—a design problem—the intensity of resource use for training and supervision, or the ratio of field staff to population, may not be enough to allow quality services; and monitoring and evaluation may not focus on this issue (chapter 4). In addition, program experience suggests that bureaucratic, professional, and political resistance to change has been underestimated. Development partners can help by:

- Giving more attention to and financial and technical assistance for improving program design, monitoring, evaluation, and management.

- Providing technical support for cost-effectiveness analysis to identify issues of intensity of resource use and providing finance for resolving them.
- Providing coordinated support and guidance on overcoming bureaucratic and political resistance to change in program strategies and design.

Addressing mismatches between causes and interventions. Three common mismatches between needs and design, outlined in chapter 3, are the "food-first" mismatch, wherein countries spend large resources on food or feeding programs when the problem lies elsewhere; the age-targeting mismatch, wherein countries invest in older children, when most malnutrition happens at younger ages; and the poverty-targeting mismatch, wherein programs fail to target malnutrition in the poorest areas, either by design or by faulty targeting. Such mismatches must be fixed if any effect is to be expected from several existing large-scale nutrition programs. Similarly, as PRSPs become important policy tools, attention must be paid to ensuring that the strategies and actions proposed in country PRSPs match the epidemiology of malnutrition in that country. Development partners can help by supporting policy analysis that identifies mismatches (see, for example, Gragnolati and others forthcoming and Shekar and Lee 2005) and with technical support and financing to help countries reorient their investments more productively.

Building commitment and capacity

Scaling up nutrition programs in countries that have underinvested and reorienting ineffective programs in countries that have invested requires strong commitment and specific institutional capacities. These two efforts also require a very specific investment in skills for building consensus among stakeholders at global and national levels.

Building commitment. Commitment building takes place in a largely unsystematic way rather than being treated as a recognized field of professional practice as important to nutrition as epidemiologic or economic analysis. It needs to be professionalized, drawing on skills from the fields of strategic communication, political and policy analysis, and organizational behavior.[4] Well-informed nutrition champions need to work systematically to:

- Build local partnerships of individuals and institutions that can influence politicians, implementing agencies, and development partners to press for increased budgets for the right kinds of nutrition investments because development partners can put more money into nutrition only if countries demand it.
- Identify gaps in the country's capacity to build commitment to improving nutrition and seek help to fill those gaps from local institutions, other

developing countries, or nongovernmental organizations (NGOs) and other development partners.

Systematic commitment-building activities can cost several hundred thousand dollars per country,[5] costs that are largely incurred before government or donor finance is available for the resulting programs or reforms. Development partners could help countries cover these costs by raising a grant fund that countries can draw on to pay for technical assistance and the upstream costs of building commitment and stakeholder consensus. To advance the state-of-the-art, they could help develop best practices and document them in a toolkit.

Building capacity. Evaluation shows that several aspects of institutional capacity building have received little attention (chapter 4). Countries need to focus more on increasing accountability to managers and clients, on improving governance, and on other measures that give implementers stronger incentives to perform. While many capacities can be strengthened during program implementation, countries need to focus also on developing capacities required before major programs are scaled up or reoriented, such as the capacities to:

- Systematically strengthen commitment.
- Analyze the relative cost-effectiveness of nutrition investments and service delivery approaches.
- Identify appropriate institutional arrangements through careful analysis of the best implementation arrangements and their fiscal and political implications.
- Develop evaluation plans and carry out quality baseline studies needed for evaluation.

Development partners could support this agenda by developing guidelines for assessing and strengthening institutional capacity, and by providing funding and technical assistance in these areas where it is needed.

Where to Focus Actions against Malnutrition

Prioritizing countries for nutrition actions

Many countries deserve priority action, given the scale of their malnutrition problems. But epidemiological considerations are only one of four key criteria for determining investment priorities across countries. The three remaining criteria are commitment, capacity, readiness for action, and to some extent, population size.

A matrix for prioritizing nutrition actions (figure 5.2) has two purposes:

- First, the matrix uses available epidemiological data to make the case that the malnutrition problem is pervasive in many countries and should therefore be an impetus for action; countries with the highest malnutrition rates in each region should be prioritized for action, followed by those with lower rates.
- Second, the matrix suggests that the response should be tailored to the magnitude and the nature of the problem. For example, where problems of underweight or stunting are overwhelming, that should be the focus of action. Where the undernutrition problem is confined to micronutrient deficiencies, those should be the focus for action. Where undernutrition issues are large and the overweight problem is emerging, actions must be targeted to both, without compromising investments in either. For overweight it may be best to scale up slowly, starting with only a few countries, to allow fine-tuning of strategies and approaches.

The detailed methods for identifying priority countries for support are outlined in technical annex 5.5. More details on regional and national epidemiology are included in technical annex 5.6.

Priority countries for nutrition actions

Three categories of countries are identified in figure 5.2, based on this classification:

- Category A: Countries that have either underweight or stunting rates greater than 20 percent.
- Category B: Countries that have either vitamin A deficiency greater than 10 percent or iron deficiency anemia prevalence greater than 20 percent.
- Category C: Countries that have an emerging overweight problem.

The matrix shows that undernutrition (both macro- and micronutrient deficiencies) and overweight are significant public health problems in most developing countries: 80 of 126 countries for which we had data fall in category A, and all 80 countries with micronutrient data fall in category B; 63 countries have both macro- and micronutrient deficiency problems (overlap between categories A and B). In about half the countries with overweight data, more than 3 percent of children are overweight (category C), and about 40 percent of these countries have both underweight and overweight problems (overlap between categories A and C), suggesting that both ends of the malnutrition spectrum (underweight and overweight) coexist in many developing countries.

Almost all the countries in the Middle East and North Africa, as expected, have both macro- and micronutrient deficiency problems that require interventions. It is also evident that overweight among children is fast becoming a public health problem even though absolute levels are still considerably low compared with the magnitude of the undernutrition problem. About one-third of the countries with overweight data have overweight prevalence rates higher than 3 percent among preschool children.

In East Asia and the Pacific, more than 70 percent of countries with data have underweight or stunting problems. Countries such as Indonesia and Mongolia carry the double burden of undernutrition and overweight problems, and the overweight problem is emerging in China.

Prevalence of undernutrition is much lower in Europe and Central Asia, but a quarter of the countries still have a stunting problem. Uzbekistan and Albania also show more than 10 percent wasting. Unsurprisingly, overweight is common; two-thirds of countries with data have an overweight problem. Besides vitamin A deficiency and iron deficiency anemia, iodine deficiency disorders (IDD) of public health significance are found in two-thirds of countries with data.

Countries in the Middle East and North Africa have a similar malnutrition profile to those in Latin America and the Caribbean. Although underweight is very limited (primarily to the Republic of Yemen), about one-third of the countries have stunting, and Djibouti has a concurrent problem of wasting. Overweight is of particular concern in the Middle East and North Africa; in all seven countries with data, more than 3 percent of children are overweight. Prevalence of overweight is higher than 5 percent in Algeria, Egypt, Jordan, and Morocco. And the high prevalence of both macro- and micronutrient deficiency in Yemen calls for immediate attention.

Although only one country in Latin America and the Caribbean region (Guatemala) shows an underweight prevalence of more then 20 percent, one-third of the countries have a problem with stunting. Vitamin A deficiency and iron deficiency anemia are also common, although the prevalence of IDD is relatively low. Overweight is pervasive in seven countries—Argentina, Bolivia, Chile, Costa Rica, Jamaica, Peru, and Uruguay—with rates of more than 5 percent.

Figure 2.12 and Maps 1.1–1.4 give additional regional and country information.

Although in South Asia overweight is currently limited to two countries, Afghanistan and Pakistan, undernutrition is incomparably high in all countries in the region; even Sri Lanka, with an under-five mortality rate of less than 20 per 1,000 live births, has about 30 percent underweight and 20 percent stunting. All countries in South Asia also have extremely high rates of vitamin A deficiency and iron deficiency anemia.

Figure 5.2 Typology and magnitude of malnutrition in World Bank regions and countries

| Category A | Stunting (20% and/or Underweight (20%) |

| VAD (10%) and/or IDA (20%) | Category B |

AFR
Côte d'Ivoire
Sâo Tomé & Principe
Somalia
Sudan

EAP
Malaysia
Solomon Islands
Timor-Leste
Vanuatu

ECA
Albania

LAC
Ecuador
St. Vincent & Grenadines

MNA
Djibouti
Iraq

SAR
Maldives
Sri Lanka

AFR
Angola
Benin
Botswana
Burkina Faso
Burundi
Cameroon
CAR
Chad
Congo, DR
Congo, Rep.
Eritrea
Ethiopia
Gabon
Ghana
Guinea
Guinea-Bissau

Lesotho
Liberia
Madagascar
Mali
Mauritania
Mozambique
Niger
Rwanda
Senegal
Sierra Leone
Swaziland
Tanzania
Togo
Uganda

EAP
Cambodia
Lao, PDR

Myanmar
Papua New Guinea
Philippines
Vietnam

ECA
Kyrgyz Rep
Tajikistan
Turkmenistan

LAC
Haiti
Honduras
Nicaragua

SAR
Bangladesh
Bhutan
India
Nepal

AFR
Gambia

EAP
Thailand

ECA
Georgia
Turkey

LAC
Dominican Rep
El Salvador

MNA
Lebanon
Syrian Arab Rep

AFR
Comoros

EAP
Kiribati

AFR
Kenya
Malawi
Namibia
Nigeria
South Africa
Zambia
Zimbabwe

EAP
Indonesia
Mongolia

ECA
Uzbekistan

LAC
Bolivia
Guatemala
Peru

MNA
Morocco
Yemen

SAR
Afghanistan
Pakistan

ECA
Armenia
Azerbaijan
Kazakhstan

LAC
Brazil
Chile
Paraguay
Venezuela

MNA
Egypt
Iran

AFR
Mauritius
Seychelles

EAP
China

ECA
Croatia
Czech Rep
Macedonia, FYR

LAC
Argentina
Costa Rica
Jamaica

Mexico
Panama
Trinidad & Tobago
Uruguay

MNA
Algeria
Jordan
Tunisia

| Category C | Overweight (3%) |

Source: WHO (2004); UNICEF and MI (2004b); De Onis and Blossner (2000).
Note: IDA = iron deficiency anemia only; VAD = vitamin A deficiency only; S = stunting only; U = underweight only; (S) = stunting with no underweight data; (U) = underweight with no stunting data; Δ = wasting; π = total goiter rate greater than 20 percent. All countries with only macronutrient deficiency do not have micronutrient information. ™ = no overweight data. AFR = Africa; EAP = East Asia and Pacific; ECA = Europe and Central Asia; LAC = Latin America and the Caribbean; MNA = Middle East and North Africa; SAR = South Asia.

Implications for action

Decisions to prioritize nutrition actions in regions and countries must be based on two criteria:

• The nature and magnitude of the nutrition problem in the region or country, as identified in the prioritization matrix.
• Country capacity, commitment, and readiness for nutrition actions, including institutional arrangements for nutrition.

Where the need is great, but capacity and commitment are low, investing in building commitment and capacity and identifying an appropriate institutional home for nutrition may be the first priority, perhaps through the vehicle of a traditional project. Where the need is high and there is some experience, commitment, and capacity for implementing nutrition actions, efforts may be best directed at scaling up pilot interventions through newer approaches and instruments, such as SWAps and PRSCs. For countries that fall in the middle of this continuum, a carefully balanced approach may be called for.

Supporting a Focused Action Research Agenda in Nutrition

Though some technical challenges remain (especially in overweight and in links between nutrition and NCDs and nutrition and HIV), there is broad consensus in the international nutrition community on many technical approaches for improving nutrition.[6] The emerging research challenges are therefore not so much technical or academic as operational, and so need to be pursued through learning-by-doing in the real world in three areas:

• Mainstreaming nutrition in the development agenda.
• Strengthening nutrition service delivery.
• Continuing to build the evidence base for how to tackle some forms of malnutrition operationally.

Research in the last area is needed to meet the rapidly growing challenge of overweight and obesity and the links between nutrition and HIV, as well as low birthweight reduction where operational experience is insufficient to scale up with confidence.

Pulling together the knowledge gaps identified earlier in the report suggests a set of action research priorities for discussion (table 5.1). Ensuring a strategic link and a synergy between the global research agenda and the global programmatic agenda—so that each drives the other—is critical for

Table 5.1 Suggested priorities for action research in nutrition

Theme	Key action research issues
Mainstreaming nutrition in the development agenda	• Mainstreaming nutrition into sector programs and PRSPs/PRSCs—how this can best be operationalized in different country circumstances. • How best to strengthen commitment to nutrition, build stakeholder consensus, and overcome resistance to change in different country circumstances. • How best to assess and build institutional capacity for nutrition policy analysis and investment planning at the country level. • Costing, financing, and institutional options for nutrition service delivery, including human resource options for nutrition services.
Strengthening and fine-tuning service delivery mechanisms	• Exploring replicability of new service delivery mechanisms in different resource-poor settings: conditional cash transfers, NGO service delivery, public-private partnerships for micronutrients, and so on. • Micronutrients: the complementary role for supplementation, fortification, and food-based strategies (including the efficacy and effectiveness of emerging technologies for food-based approaches such as biofortification). • Targeting and cost-effectiveness of food supplementation linked to nutrition education and growth promotion to maximize the effect on the mother-child dyad.
Further strengthening the evidence base for what works operationally	• Evidence-based strategies to prevent and reduce overweight and diet-related NCDs. • Efficacy and effectiveness of nutrition interventions in HIV programs, such as the role of exclusive breastfeeding in preventing mother-to-child transmission in developing countries; the role of food security in preventing HIV; and the role of nutrition in enhancing the effectiveness of antiretroviral therapy. • Linking nutrition data with larger global monitoring initiatives such as the Health Metrics Network and other MDG and poverty monitoring initiatives, such as the national sample surveys, Multiple-Indicator Cluster Surveys, Demographic and Health Surveys, and Living Standards Measurement Surveys. • Methodologies for evaluating nutrition in the context of programmatic approaches (SWAps and PRSCs); fine-tuning the indicators—are we setting higher standards for nutrition than for other sectors?

Note: For details, see annex 3.

future investments in nutrition to succeed. Development partners could help countries pursue these priorities by providing funds and technical assistance for designing the action research and documenting, evaluating, and disseminating results. Further details on suggested action research priorities appear in annex 3.

The Gaps between Identified Needs and Development Partners' Focus

The development community, and the world as a whole, has consistently failed to address malnutrition over the past decades. The consequences of failure to act on what has been long known about how malnutrition undermines economic growth and perpetuates poverty are now evident in the slow progress toward the MDGs. The unequivocal choice now is between acting on what has been known for so long or continuing to fail.

Few development partners have clear nutrition policies or strategies. The main gaps between the operational needs for scaling up and the focus of development partners lie in four areas:

- Mainstreaming undernutrition and micronutrient programs, as well as integrating nutrition into HIV/AIDS programs.
- Identifying strategies for addressing the emerging epidemic of obesity and building the evidence base for the link between early undernutrition and later susceptibility to NCDs, as well as diet-related NCDs.
- Building commitment.
- Identifying workable institutional arrangements for, and developing institutional capacity in promoting, managing, monitoring, and evaluating large-scale nutrition actions.

The World Bank is the largest investor in global nutrition, with many other investments in its portfolio that can improve nutrition more generally. However, it will take several decades for many of its investments to improve nutrition adequately. Given the magnitude of the problem (chapter 2), the Bank's investments in direct interventions (short route) are extremely small—not more than 3.8 percent of its lending for human development and less than 0.7 percent of Bank-wide lending in 2000–4.

Currently, only 36 Bank-supported investments include some direct support for nutrition. The Bank's total investment is $662 million, spread across Health, Nutrition, and Population (22 investments); Agriculture and Rural Development (5); Education (4); Social Protection (3); and Transport (2 emergency rehabilitation projects). Most of these investments are less than $10 million and only nine have somewhat more substantive (albeit modest) investments in Argentina, Bangladesh, Eritrea, India and its state of Andhra

Pradesh, Iran, Madagascar, Senegal, and Uganda. Yet undernutrition is serious in more than 80 developing countries. The gap between the need and the level of investment, paralleled in the efforts of other development partners, is indeed very large.

Next Steps

The next steps address the gaps between current focus and identified needs in scaling up nutrition actions at global and country levels.

At the global level, the development community needs to unite in explicitly recognizing the role of malnutrition as an underlying cause of mortality, morbidity, and slow economic growth in countries, and to agree on five next steps:

- Coordinating efforts to strengthen commitment, consensus, and funding for nutrition within global and country-level partnerships such as the Child Survival Partnership, the Partnership for Safe Motherhood and Neonatal Health, the New Partnership for Africa's Development (NEPAD), GAIN, SCN, the Micronutrient Initiative (MI), national and global alliances, and public-private partnerships.
- Agreeing on broad strategic priorities for the next decade (such as the three operational priorities and three research themes proposed above) and applying their comparative advantage to each area.
- Agreeing on priority countries for investing in nutrition and for mainstreaming and scaling up nutrition programs (see figure 5.2, figure 2.2, and maps 1–4).
- Agreeing on priority countries for testing systematic approaches to mainstreaming nutrition, building commitment and capacity, and reducing overweight and obesity.
- Making a collective effort to switch financing from small-scale projects to large-scale programs, except where small projects with strong monitoring and evaluation components are required to pilot-test interventions and delivery systems.

In addition, the grant development agencies and foundations need to work together to make funding available at global and national levels to promote and finance the country commitment and capacity-building activities needed before large-scale investments or program reforms are made. Development partners should also encourage well-designed action research on large-scale nutrition programs and more systematic monitoring and evaluation so we can learn from this research and share the resulting knowledge internationally. The World Bank has recently committed to support the International Centre for Diarrhoeal Disease Research, Bangladesh

(ICDDR,B) through a small catalytic development grant ($3.6 million) that will allow ICDDR,B to undertake such activities. Development partners need to strategize together to see how this model can be a catalyst for additional investments to empower other global and regional agencies to play a similar stepped-up role.

At the country level, the development community needs to agree on four next steps:

• In all countries with micronutrient deficiencies, develop a national strategy for micronutrients, finance it, and scale up micronutrient programs to nationwide coverage within five years. An important caveat: while we strongly endorse the need to take the micronutrients agenda to completion, it must not crowd out the need for attention to general undernutrition, as has been the experience in several countries and agencies over the past decade.
• In all countries with undernutrition and overweight problems, in the medium or shorter term:
  – Identify and support at least five to ten countries with large nutrition problems where development partners collectively work toward mainstreaming nutrition into SWAps, Multi-country AIDS Projects (MAPs), and PRSCs (as in Bangladesh and in Madagascar). Where countries have little experience with such investments, nutrition projects may be the first step toward building capacity.
  – Identify and support at least three to five countries where existing large-scale investments can be reoriented to maximize impact. In these countries, provide constructive and coordinated technical support to reorient program design and strengthen implementation quality.
  – Identify and support at least three to five countries where nutrition issues loom large, but where limited investment is available (as in Ethiopia). In these countries, invest in building commitment and provide technical support to develop coordinated strategies that can then be financed through complementary resources from development partners.[7]

The challenge—especially in low-income developing countries—will be to take the unfinished micronutrient agenda to completion and slowly introduce attention and tested strategies to address the overweight agenda, without crowding out attention, capacity, and funding for the most important undernutrition agenda. Initial estimates suggest that the costs for addressing the micronutrient agenda in Africa will be approximately $235 million a year. Costs for other regions and for other aspects of the nutrition agenda have yet to be estimated. Other gross estimates are much larger,

($750 million for global costs for two doses of Vitamin A supplementation per year; between $1 billion and $1.5 billion for global salt iodization, including $800 million to $1.2 billion leveraged from the private sector; and several billion dollars for community nutrition programs).[8] A more detailed costing exercise is being conducted by the World Bank to come up with realistic figures.

One way to prioritize the selection of these countries and actions is to use the tools outlined here and in technical annexes 5.4, 5.5, and 5.6, while considering country capacity, commitment, and readiness for action. The balance between long and short route interventions (identified in chapter 3) will be critical. The agenda proposed here needs to be debated, modified, agreed on, funded, and acted on in concert by development partners through a process of consultation and dissemination.

Notes

1. Pelletier, Shekar, and Du (forthcoming).

2. Pelletier, Shekar, and Du (forthcoming); Habicht, Victora, and Vaughan (1999).

3. Most development partners share the health sector bias. In UNICEF, USAID, and the World Bank, for example, nutrition is managed by the agencies' health bureaus. Of 36 current World Bank-supported projects that include nutrition, 22 are in the health sector, the other 14 in agriculture and rural development (5), education (4), social protection (3) and transport (2) (from April 2005 Portfolio review).

4. Heaver (2005b).

5. Heaver (2005b).

6. *Lancet* series on child survival (2004).

7. In doing this, several steps may be involved:

- Helping countries identify the local causes of malnutrition, and malnutrition's importance compared with other development constraints.
- Helping with practical tools for deciding how to invest (see technical annex 5.4).
- Helping develop a national intervention strategy and a matching action research program.
- Putting in place the public expenditure reorientation needed to finance the strategy.
- Agreeing on a cofinancing strategy that makes best use of each development partner's comparative advantages (technical support, financing, monitoring and evaluation, and on-the ground presence).

8. Hunt (2005).

Annex 1
Country Experience with Short Routes to Improving Nutrition

Intervention	Large-scale program experience	Effect on nutrition*	Costs per participant per year[a]	Best practices
Community-based growth promotion	Indonesia UPGK; Tamil Nadu Integrated Nutrition Program; BINP; Madagascar SEECALINE; Nicaragua PROCOSAN (Health Sector Reform Project; Honduras AIN-C (national); Tanzania Iringa; Thailand National Nutrition	+	$1.60–$1 0.00 recurrent additional budgetary cost; $11–$18 if food added	Target to children under age two. Tailored, negotiated, two-way counseling with mother; messages based on "trials of improved practices"; can integrate preventive health and rapid response to danger signals and mental stimulation. Medical and nursing personnel need training and motivation to support.
Vitamin A supplements (to preschool children)	India, Indonesia, Bangladesh, Ghana, Nepal, Pakistan, Niger, Tanzania, Senegal	+	$1.01–$2.55	Campaign approach needs perennial motivation and mobilization. Need to integrate into mainstream medical services. Medical and nursing personnel need training.
Vitamin A fortification	Guatemala (sugar)	+	$.69–$.98 per high risk person reached	Special attention to regulatory enforcement of fortification laws to ensure industry compliance; consumer education may be needed; costs are usually small and can often be passed on to consumers, except when a targeted subsidy is warranted.

Intervention	Large-scale program experience	Effect on nutrition*	Costs per participant per year[a]	Best practices
Iron supplementation (daily to pregnant women, _, and children under age two, C)	Indonesia _ Thailand _ Cuba _, C Bolivia _, C Honduras AIN-C C Zambia C Nicaragua PRO-COSAN C	+	$.55–$3.17	Counseling to address resistance points and motivations needed; reminders enhance adherence; medical and nursing staff need to be educated and motivated; consider combining with community-based growth promotion.
Iron fortification	Venezuela, United States, Canada, United Kingdom, Sweden, Chile	+	$.12–$.22	Special attention to regulatory enforcement of fortification laws to ensure industry compliance; consumer education may be needed; costs are usually small and can often be passed on to consumers, except when a targeted subsidy is warranted.
Salt iodization	China Salt Iodization Project; Indonesia Iodine Project Worldwide	+	$.20–$.50	Special attention needed to regulatory enforcement of fortification laws; consumer education may be needed. Consolidation of alternative employment for artisan producers. Costs are usually small and can often be passed on to consumers.
Conditional cash transfers	Mexico PROGRESA Honduras PRAF Nicaragua Red de Protección Social (RPS)	+/-	$70–$77	Pay attention to the quality of nutrition counseling in health services. Consider combining with community-based growth promotion.

Intervention	Large-scale program experience	Effect on nutrition*	Costs per participant per year[a]	Best practices
Maternal-child food supplementation (listed countries have NGO programs evaluated for impact)	Ethiopia, Gambia, Kenya, Benin, Madagascar, Mozambique, India, Bolivia, Guatemala, Haiti, Peru, Honduras, Nicaragua Virtually every country.	+/-	$42 per 1,000 calories per day per person	Tight targeting critical. Important that food not be disincentive to family or local agriculture; nutrition education critical; avoid foreign foods, use local foods if possible; targeting to malnourished risks rewarding failure.
Early child development/Child care	Bolivia PIDI Colombia HBI Uganda ECD India ICDS Philippines ECD Kenya ECD	+/-	$250–$412 with food (Colombia, Bolivia); $2–$3 without food (Uganda)	Involve parents in growth promotion and child development through interpersonal counseling and community meetings.
Nutrition education (breastfeeding promotion, complementary feeding)	Most small nutrition components and information, education, and communication in health-based nutrition projects.	+/-	$2.50	Most common problem is poorly designed messages, materials, and media. Counseling messages should be tailored, negotiated, and based on formative research in the community. Generic information, education, and communication and group talks ineffective.
Breastfeeding promotion in hospitals	Brazil, Honduras, Mexico Baby-friendly hospitals	+	$.30–$.40 if infant formula in ward $2–$3 if no infant formula in ward	For hospital-based births; education of medical and nursing professional critical, as is keeping infant formula purveyors out of hospitals.

Intervention	Large-scale program experience	Effect on nutrition*	Costs per participant per year[a]	Best practices
Microcredit cum nutrition education	Ghana Bolivia Uganda	+	$.90–$3.50 (marginal cost of nutrition education)	Freedom from Hunger (NGO). Pay attention to quality of nutrition counseling.
Facility-based integrated nutrition services such as IMCI (micro-nutrient supplements, growth monitoring, nutrition education, prenatal nutrition; care of severely malnourished)	Honduras AIN		—	Educating medical and nursing personnel about breastfeeding, infant feeding, growth, and micronutrients is essential.

— = not available.

a. Costing is a complex exercise, and the costs presented here, extracted from several sources, are not necessarily comparable. We include the information here simply to emphasize the point that costing is important in setting priorities.

Annex 2
Long Routes to Improving Nutrition

Economic growth

Economic growth is perhaps the most important long route to improved nutrition. Although nutrition is correlated with income, both across countries and over time in the same country, improvement takes a long time—time during which many children suffer irreparable damage to human capital. Haddad and others (2002) estimate that countries with 2.5 percent GDP growth per capita could expect a reduction of 27 percent in underweight in preschool children between 1990 and 2015.

Macroeconomic policies

Macroeconomic policies, particularly trade policies, can profoundly affect both the supply of and the demand for food. Policy reforms can have a rapid effect on the income of the poor, but their effect on nutrition is less direct, and pro-poor reforms have often proven to be politically difficult to implement. As was shown in the Sahel in 1996 when the CFA franc was devalued, foreign exchange rates have an immediate and large effect on food consumption of the rich and poor alike. Unfortunately, government controls on food markets (tariffs, subsidies, price controls, ration shops, public ownership of mills, and parastatal food marketing boards) often fail to benefit the poor, while draining the public coffers.[1] Reforms of such programs can improve poor people's nutrition or food consumption and reduce public expenditures (usually by reducing benefits to wealthy and politically powerful populations, however). Careful food policy analysis on the effect of policy changes on food consumption of the poor can show which policy reforms make the most sense. A good example of this type of analysis is Romania's Agricultural Sector Adjustment Loan;[2] it identified the regressiveness of food subsidies and tariffs, and at the same time built local capacity to undertake food policy analysis.

Female education and enhanced women's status

Female education and enhancing the status of women are important long routes to nutritional improvement.[3] In a large cross-country study, women's education was found to have a greater influence on child nutrition than food availability, women's status, and access to safe water.[4] Improving women's education and status is desirable for many reasons, of course, but the lag time between girls entering school and having their first child (hopefully delayed by additional schooling) and the slow pace of improvement in women's status make these long-term approaches to improving nutrition. In Ethiopia, analysis showed that increased schooling, food security, and income growth would take too long to affect preschool malnutrition, but that community-based growth promotion could accelerate and potentiate their effect on nutrition.[5] The nutritional effect of growth promotion among 25 percent of children is equivalent to primary schooling in one female adult per household. This had been shown previously in the Bank-supported Indonesian Nutrition Development Project, where growth promotion was shown to have the greatest effect on mothers with the least education.[6]

Women's workload

Women's workload is also important for nutrition. Women are farmers and wage workers, and they carry out the bulk of family maintenance (cooking, washing, child care). Women's income can have an important positive effect on child nutrition, if child-care arrangements are adequate. Relieving this workload through labor-saving devices (food mills, wheelbarrows, improved stoves, water supply) can free both time and energy for attention to nutrition, both for the woman and her children. Many development programs expect women to "do more" for health when they have no time available. Attention to women's income, control of resources, energy expenditure, and time use is critical to improving the nutrition of women and children.

Food production

Food production is also a long route to nutrition improvement. Countries with higher food availability tend to have better nutrition. Nonetheless, nutrition does not track food availability within countries over time. This is undoubtedly because those who need the food the most are unlikely to be able to increase production or purchasing power in the short term, unless explicit efforts are made to increase their economic access to food. Also, as shown in studies of agricultural commercialization by the International

Food Policy Research Institute,[7] the effect of income on nutrition is mediated by women's control of income and their time.[8]

Water supply and sanitation

Diarrhea, a major cause of malnutrition, is strongly related to water access and quality,[9] so it is not surprising that water supply and sanitation have been shown to have an effect on nutrition.[10] Water supply programs not only reduce the waterborne transmission of disease, but also save women time and energy otherwise spent carrying water. This extra time can be devoted to child care and feeding or to income generation, and the extra energy benefits undernourished women. Water and sanitation programs might find that their cost-benefit increases if they measure their effect on improving nutrition.

Family planning

The relationship between nutrition and fertility is complex. On the one hand, exclusive breastfeeding (arguably the most important nutrition intervention) reduces fertility. On the other hand, high parity and short birth intervals are associated with worse child nutrition and maternal nutritional depletion. Family planning affects nutrition both by enhancing maternal resources available to each child and by enhancing women's health. Such programs rarely measure nutrition as an outcome, but a successful family planning program is likely to have a substantial positive effect on nutrition. Thus maternal health and family planning programs provide another long route to nutritional improvement.

Notes

1. Alderman and Lindert (1998); Adams (1998); Tuck and Lindert (1996); World Bank (2001c).
2. Esanu and Lindert (1996).
3. Smith and others (2003); women's status is proxied by whether women work for cash, age at first marriage, age difference between partners, and education difference between partners.
4. Smith and Haddad (2000).
5. Christiaensen and Alderman (2004).
6. Manoff International, Inc. (1984).
7. Von Braun (1995).
8. Haddad and others (1996).
9. Cairncross and Valdimanis (2004).
10. Anderson (1981); Burger and Esrey (1995).

11. Heaver (2002).
12. Monteiro and others (2004).
13. Panneth and Susser (1995).
14. Caballero (2005).

Annex 3
Key Priorities for Action Research in Nutrition: A Proposal

Mainstreaming Nutrition in the Development Agenda

A new programming environment is emerging at the global and country levels. The move from projects to programs, from vertical, disease-specific approaches to sectorwide approaches (SWAps), and budget support are all part of this changing picture. The roles of civil society and the private sector are becoming more important in global health and nutrition. The focus on results has never been higher on the agenda of development partners. These changes call for some adjustments in how the nutrition agenda is furthered. Four key areas of action research are critical in making these adjustments:

- *Mainstreaming nutrition into health, agriculture, rural development, education, and social protection programs.* As outlined in chapter 1, evidence now shows that several of the health and other Millennium Development Goals (MDGs) will not be met without investments in improving nutrition. Some evidence suggests that nutrition education efforts and other demand-side interventions may be necessary but not sufficient to improve outcomes unless these efforts are linked to supply-side interventions such as improved access to health services and micronutrient supplementation and fortification, supplementary feeding, and increased access to cheaper fruits and vegetables for addressing overweight. Programs across many sectors have attempted to include nutrition interventions. Yet very little information is available on how best to do so or which approaches are successful. The Bank-supported development grant for the International Centre for Diarrhoeal Disease Research, Bangladesh (ICDDR,B) will look at opportunities to include nutrition in maternal and child health programs. There is a need to review and support similar experiences in other sectors.

• *Guidelines and instruments for assessing institutional capacity.* As outlined in chapter 4, a key constraint on action in nutrition is the institutional arrangements and capacity for nutrition.[11] Many programs are unsuccessful because not enough effort is invested in assessing capacities and in defining capacity needs. Developing guidelines and instruments for assessing institutional capacity and identifying best practices for institutional arrangements in different country scenarios will be critical to helping countries make rational assessments for scaling up programs. Human resource options for nutrition service delivery under different institutional arrangements and their management and fiscal implications need to be researched.

• *Building commitment for nutrition.* How should these commitment-building approaches vary in different country circumstances, and how can international and local stakeholders best partner to strengthen commitment?

• *Costing and financing interventions and service delivery approaches in varied country circumstances.* The Copenhagen Consensus (Behrman, Alderman, and Hoddinott 2004) has shown that nutrition interventions rank very high among other interventions in terms of cost-benefit. While some information is available for costing individual interventions, very little is available on large-scale programs and the levels of investments needed to meet the nutrition MDGs.

Strengthening and Fine-Tuning Delivery Mechanism

• *Exploring the replicability of new delivery mechanisms for nutrition services.* Where government capacities for implementation are limited, countries have explored service delivery through nongovernmental organizations (NGOs), as in Bangladesh. Lessons suggest that this may warrant an alternative capacity for contracting and managing NGOs. In other countries (such as Mexico and Honduras), conditional cash transfers have been used as an opportunity for strengthening the use of health and nutrition services. In the micronutrient sector, public-private partnerships and alliances are being explored. Experience and learning from these innovations needs to be tested in other environments for future adaptation and scaling-up.

• *Research to support a clearer understanding of how far micronutrient supplementation can take us (and for which micronutrients), how long it should be continued under different conditions, and whether fortification or food-based strategies are sufficient.* The efficacy of biofortification and other emerging food-based strategies for micronutrient deficiency control is being explored through initiatives such as the Harvest Plus program. These strategies have immense potential that must be maximized.

- *Cost-effectiveness of food supplementation (linked to nutrition education), and conditions under which costs may outweigh potential benefits.* Food supplementation often consumes 50 percent or more of program budgets. Evidence suggests that to be effective, food supplementation must be linked to nutrition education through growth promotion or other strategies, especially for young children. Yet the evidence is unclear as to what the best targeting mechanisms are and when costs may outweigh benefits.
- *Devise methodologies for forging stakeholder consensus* around results from operations research and monitoring and evaluation as well as the programmatic vision and capacities to fine-tune strategies based on these inputs.

Strengthening the Evidence Base:

- *Evidence-based strategies to prevent and reduce overweight and diet-related noncommunicable diseases (NCDs).* This is a key challenge because it affects both rich and poor countries; these problems contribute substantially to chronic disease and mortality, as well as to economic growth; and reversing overweight offers huge public expenditure savings in both low-income and middle-income countries. The poor in low socioeconomic status countries (gross national product [GNP] less than $2,500 per capita) may be protected against obesity, but the poor in upper middle-income countries (GNP greater than $2,500 per capita) are much more prone to obesity.[12] In addition, the Barker hypothesis suggests that fetal food deprivation may result in postnatal programming that predisposes low-birthweight babies to cardiovascular disease and diabetes.[13] Furthermore, in many areas obesity coexists with underweight.[14] However, precise information on the size and scope of the overweight problem as well as the diet-NCD link and tested large-scale interventions on how to address them are still limited. Therefore, the priority here is to find out more about these issues as we move toward scaling up.
- *Efficacy and effectiveness of different nutrition interventions for preventing and mitigating the effect of HIV/AIDS.* These interventions include the role of exclusive breastfeeding in preventing mother-to-child transmission of HIV/AIDS; the role of nutrition in enhancing the effectiveness of antiretroviral therapy; and the role of food security in mitigating the risk of HIV infection.

- *Linking nutrition data with larger global monitoring initiatives.* Several larger global health and poverty monitoring initiatives (such as the Health Metrics Network) are under development. Development partners and funding agencies are keen to support integrated systems, and it is important that relevant nutrition indicators be included in these initiatives. This will need some research support.
- *Methodologies for evaluating nutrition actions in the context of programmatic approaches such as SWAps and Poverty Reduction Strategy Credits (PRSC)s.* The current evaluation methodologies may need to be adjusted and adapted to these new approaches. In addition, the indicators that are used for assessing progress in nutrition are much harder to apply than those in other sectors. For example, the MDG progress indicator for the education sector is school enrollment rates. The nutrition indicator is underweight rates. While the education indicator is much closer to being a process or output indicator, the nutrition indicator is much more of an impact indicator—and the time frame for achieving an impact in underweight is much longer than that for enrolling children in school. In the choice of indicators, we may be setting nutrition up for higher standards than other sectors. This issue needs some research. In addition, many traditional nutrition evaluations have looked for the benefits of programs across population groups as whole—for example, low-birthweight prevention programs have looked for an impact among all pregnant women. However, emerging research has shown that these benefits may be unequally distributed across different groups (for example, the poorest or the most malnourished may benefit more), or that benefits may be distributed differently across the mother-child dyad under different situations—yet the evaluation methodology used often limits the size and nature of the benefits that can be detected.

Technical Annexes

Annex 1.1
Ten selected risk factors of major burden of disease

Developing countries with high child and high or very high adult mortality[a]		*Developing countries with low child and low adult mortality*[b]		*Developed countries with very low or low child mortality levels*[c]	
Risk factor	*% DALYs*	*Risk factor*	*% DALYs*	*Risk factor*	*% DALYs*
1 Underweight	14.9	Alcohol	6.2	Tobacco	12.2
2 Unsafe sex	10.2	Blood pressure	5.0	Blood pressure	10.9
3 Unsafe water/ sanitation/hygiene	5.5	Tobacco	4.0	Alcohol	9.2
4 Indoor smoke from solid fuels	3.7	Underweight	3.1	Cholesterol	7.6
5 Zinc deficiency	3.2	Overweight	2.7	Overweight	7.4
6 Iron deficiency	3.1	Cholesterol	2.1	Low fruit and vegetable intake	3.9
7 Vitamin A deficiency	3.0	Low fruit and vegetable intake	1.9	Physical inactivity	3.3
8 Blood pressure	2.5	Indoor smoke from solid fuels	1.9	Illicit drugs	1.8
9 Tobacco	2.0	Iron deficiency	1.8	Unsafe sex	0.8
10 Cholesterol	1.9	Unsafe water/ sanitation/hygiene	1.7	Iron deficiency	0.7

Source: WHO (2002).
Note: Calculation is based on WHO regions:
[a] = AFR-D, AFR-E, AMR-D, EMR-D, SEAR-D
[b] =AMR-B, EMR-B, SEAR-B, WPR-B
[c] =AMR-A, EUR-A, EUR-B, EUR-C, WPR-A
Unsafe sex disease burden is from HIV/AIDS and sexually transmitted diseases; iron deficiency disease burden is from maternal and perinatal causes, as well as direct effects of anemia; unsafe water, sanitation, and hygiene disease burden is from diarrheal diseases.

Annex 1.2
Trends in selected development indicators in developing countries

	1970	1975	1980	1981	1984	1985	1987	1990	1993	1995	1996	1999	2000	2001	2002	2003	2005	ARC*
IMR (/1000)	108		88					71		67			62			60		-1.80
U5MR (/1000)	167		133					105		98			91			87		-1.99
Energy availability (Cal)	2110	2146	2308			2444		2520		2602			2654					0.83
Underweight (%)			37.6			33.9		30.1		27.3			24.8				22.7	-2.99
Stunting (%)			48.6			43.2		37.9		33.5			29.6				26.5	-2.03
Poverty headcount (%)				40.4	32.8		28.4	27.9	26.3		22.8	21.8		21.1				-2.45

Source: IMR & U5MR: www.childinfo.org; underweight and stunting: SCN (2004); poverty headcount: Chen and Ravallion (2004); energy availability: FAO Statistical Database (2005).

Note: IMR = infant mortality rate; U5MR = under-five mortality rate; ARC = annual rate of change; per capita energy availability is an average of three years.

Figure A.1 Trends in selected development indicators in developing countries

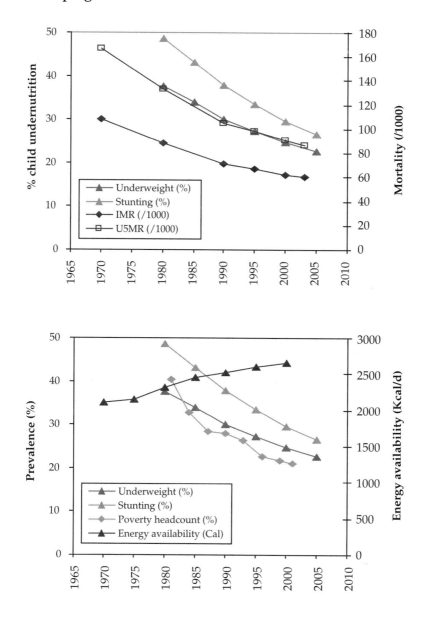

Figure A.2 Differences in aggregate per capita food availability and percent child underweight levels

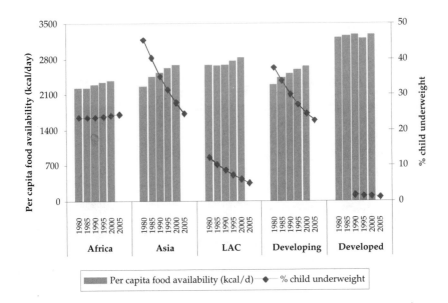

Source: SCN (2004); FAO Statistical Database (2005).

Annex 1.3
Estimated percentage reduction in prevalence of malnutrition between 1990 and 2015 and number of years to halve prevalence of malnutrition, through economic growth alone

Elasticity Econ. growth	Percentage reduction in prevalence of malnutrition, 1990–2015			No. of years to halve the prevalence of malnutrition		
	-0.3	-0.5	-0.7	-0.3	-0.5	-0.7
0.5	3.7	6.1	8.4	461.8	276.9	197.7
1.0	7.2	11.8	16.1	230.7	138.3	98.7
1.5	10.7	17.2	23.2	153.7	92.1	65.7
2.0	14.0	22.2	29.7	115.2	69.0	49.2
2.5	17.2	27.0	35.7	92.1	55.1	39.3
3.0	20.2	31.5	41.2	76.7	45.9	32.7
3.5	23.2	35.7	46.2	65.7	39.3	27.9
4.0	26.1	39.7	50.8	57.4	34.3	24.4
4.5	28.8	43.4	55.1	51.0	30.5	21.7
5.0	31.5	46.9	59.0	45.9	27.4	19.5
5.5	34.0	50.2	62.5	41.7	24.9	17.7
6.0	36.5	53.3	65.8	38.2	22.8	16.2
6.5	38.9	56.2	68.8	35.2	21.0	14.9
7.0	41.2	59.0	71.5	32.7	19.5	13.8
7.5	43.4	61.5	74.0	30.5	18.1	12.9
8.0	45.5	64.0	76.3	28.5	17.0	12.0
8.5	47.6	66.2	78.4	26.8	16.0	11.3
9.0	49.6	68.4	80.3	25.3	15.1	10.7
9.5	51.5	70.4	82.1	24.0	14.2	10.1
10.0	53.3	72.3	83.7	22.8	13.5	9.6

Source: Authors' calculation based on different per capita GDP growth (0.5 to 10.0 percent per capita per year) and elasticity assumptions (-0.3 to -0.7).

For example, in countries with an annual GDP growth of 2.5 percent per capita and an elasticity of -0.5, one can expect a 27 percent reduction in underweight rates between 1990 and 2010.

Annex 2.1
Estimated prevalence of malnutrition among preschool children by region

Stunting	1980	1985	1990	1995	2000	2005
Africa	39.0	37.8	36.9	36.1	35.2	34.5
Asia	55.1	48.2	41.1	35.4	30.1	25.7
LAC	24.3	21.1	18.3	15.9	13.7	11.8
Developing	48.6	43.2	37.9	33.5	29.6	26.5
Developed			2.8	2.8	2.7	2.6
Global			33.5	29.9	26.7	24.1

Underweight	1980	1985	1990	1995	2000	2005
Africa	23.5	23.5	23.6	23.9	24.2	24.5
Asia	45.4	40.5	35.1	31.5	27.9	24.8
LAC	12.5	10.5	8.7	7.3	6.1	5.0
Developing	37.6	33.9	30.1	27.3	24.8	22.7
Developed			1.6	1.4	1.3	1.1
Global			26.5	24.3	22.2	20.6

Overweight	1980	1985	1990	1995	2000	2005
Africa				3.3	4.2	5.2
Asia				2.6	2.5	2.5
LAC				4.4	4.3	4.3
Developing				2.9	3.0	3.4

Source: SCN (2004); de Onis (2004a).

Annex 3.1
Obesity and chronic disease in the developing world

Many developing countries are starting to parallel the developed world, with increasing prevalence of overweight and obesity and associated chronic disease comorbidities. Overweight and obesity put individuals at higher risk for dyslipidemia, hypertension, hyperinsulinism, insulin resistance, and diabetes, all of which substantially increase the risk for cardiovascular disease. Obese individuals may also suffer from respiratory disorders and certain types of cancer. In 2001, it was estimated that chronic diseases contributed to approximately 60 percent of the 56.5 million total reported deaths in the world and to approximately 46 percent of the global burden of disease. Reflecting this trend, the World Health Organization (WHO) has recently made a call to action to put overweight and obesity at the forefront of public health policies and programs.

There are many potential reasons for the strikingly high prevalence of overweight and obesity and their comorbidities in developing countries. Behavioral factors, including dietary intake, physical activity, and sedentary behaviors, have been important contributors to the development of obesity. Intakes of total fat, animal products, and sugar are increasing simultaneously with decreases in the consumption of cereals, fruits, and vegetables. Decreased energy expenditure, due to an increasingly sedentary lifestyle and a reduction in labor-intensive occupations, is a second and equally important explanation for the increased rates of overweight and obesity in the developing world. Major changes in lifestyle have occurred over the past several decades, and have caused an "obesogenic environment" because of the easy availability of high-energy food combined with an increasingly sedentary lifestyle.

Although obesity is the result of a complex interplay between genetics and environment, obesity and chronic diseases are largely preventable. There is compelling evidence for the power of societal and environmental factors to contribute to weight gain. Beyond the medical treatment necessary for the people who are already overweight or obese, there is an underutilized opportunity for primary prevention through cost-effective and sustainable interventions. Given the limited resources of the developing world in particular, it is clear that obesity prevention needs to be incorporated into existing nutrition programs. Unfortunately, little is known about the prevention and treatment of overweight and obesity on a population level, particularly in developing countries.

Interventions addressing obesity span from clinic-based, one-on-one consultations with a primary-care physician to large-scale policy or social marketing initiatives. Clinical interventions target adults and children who are already overweight or obese. There are several possibilities for clinic-based interventions, which include dietary management, exercise programs, pharmacological treatment, psychotherapy, behavior modification, and surgical treatment. Most successful programs have combined diet and exercise approaches with behavior therapy.

School-based programs are becoming increasingly popular in the United States due to the captive audience of children in the school setting. The findings from studies of school-based interventions are modest at best, and do not always sustain results over time. Workplace interventions include promotion of stair use, on-site recreational facilities and programs, incentives for active commuting to work, and physical activity and nutrition counseling. Although most worksite interventions are able to show short-term changes in behavior, in large part they are not able to assess whether any change in body mass index (BMI) or adiposity resulted from the program.

The most successful programs have taken a community-level approach, and have addressed obesity through multiple, simultaneous and different avenues. The key elements of the successful interventions include having an environmental and multidisciplinary approach; generating local adaptations of programs; exploring cultural norms and fitting the program within those constructs; adhering to a social-ecological model of behavior change; and taking a multifaceted approach to include multiple stakeholders, including health professionals, educators, and policy makers. Unfortunately, many of these types of programs have not been sufficiently evaluated. Those that have been evaluated do not always show any impact on BMI, and some have actually shown an increase in BMI across the course of the program.

A wide variety of policy interventions are possible and have achieved mixed success. Social marketing campaigns are another approach to obesity prevention, but have been shown to be only marginally successful. The programs are generally successful in raising awareness about health issues, particularly through the use of mass media and point-of-purchase promotions, multichannel marketing, and consumer-driven research. However, it is very difficult to capture any changes in individual-level behavior or health status change.

Despite the apparent, albeit moderate, effectiveness of several types of interventions, there are operational challenges that exist to addressing the problem of obesity in the developing world. The primary challenge is the lack of financing and institutional capacity to approach the problem in many developing countries. Several other political and economic issues hinder the effectiveness of interventions in developing countries. These include lack of understanding by key decision makers, such as health ministers, that obesity and chronic disease are critical issues and threats to public health; a misguided perception by policy makers that obesity is a result of personal irresponsibility and therefore outside of the domain of policy; and an assumption that global development and economic growth are the most important goals for the developing world, with disregard for the health consequences that come along with such economic growth. A related challenge is that transitional economies are facing the dual burden of undernutrition simultaneous with a high prevalence of obesity. In addition to these political and economic barriers to effective prevention and control of obesity are strong cultural and social norms working against that goal.

Large gaps in research relating to obesity prevention and management have been identified. The primary gap is the lack of high-quality evaluations of obesity prevention interventions. Another important gap in the research arena is the lack of behavioral research, including research on the environmental, familial, and societal influences on food intake and physical activity. Cost-effectiveness will certainly be enhanced through improved targeting of programs and interventions to the populations who will benefit most.

Source: Fernald (2005).

Annex 4.1
Country experiences in nutrition programming

A. India: Two approaches to food supplementation—The Tamil Nadu Integrated Nutrition Projects and the Integrated Child Development Services

India's Tamil Nadu Integrated Nutrition Program (TINP) operated in about 20,000 villages. It began in 1980, and was absorbed by the national Integrated Child Development Services Program (ICDS) in 1997. The two programs had quite different approaches to food supplementation.

TINP served children a slightly sweetened snack food early in the morning, which was seen by mothers as a supplement, rather than a meal. ICDS feeding is at lunchtime, and so substitutes for a meal at home. The ICDS timing suits older children, who can walk to the feeding center. TINP's early morning supplementation was at a time when mothers could bring children under three—the most nutritionally vulnerable—to the nutrition center before they went to work.

TINP supplemented only children who were malnourished or whose growth was faltering; they "graduated" from supplementation when their growth was back on track. ICDS feeds a specific number of children every day, who may or may not be malnourished or growth faltering. Since the same children are fed every day, food is seen as an entitlement, rather than a temporary supplement designed to get the child back on track and to show mothers how they can prevent or treat malnutrition at home by feeding small, affordable amounts of extra food.

The TINP system was both more effective in terms of reducing malnutrition, and cheaper, because an average of 25 percent of children were supplemented on a given day, in comparison to ICDS' 40 percent. But, because different children came into TINP supplementation as and when their growth faltered, 75 percent of TINP children got supplementation at different times, thus encouraging broad community acceptance of the program.

Source: Heaver (2003a).

B. Senegal: Empowering communities by involving them in the design, delivery, and management of services

In Senegal's first World Bank–supported Community Nutrition Project:

* Clients helped influence the design of services during a pilot intervention a year before the main project began. They determined what open-
ing hours for the nutrition centers best suited them. They also insisted
on more information, education, communication sessions, and themes
than the designers of the pilot had originally intended.
* The choice of community nutrition workers was approved by local steering committees representing the community, which then met their nutrition workers and their supervisor once a month to review progress.
* Community nutrition workers organized "social mobilizations"
bimonthly to keep the broader community informed about progress.
* Project clients contributed about 3 percent of the costs of running the
nutrition centers; the amount was nominal, but the principle of user
charges made the nutrition services more accountable to the community.
* During the project, communities were encouraged to analyze their local
problems and take action to deal with them. One initiative was that day-
care centers for children were started in 137 nutrition centers at the
request of and financed by the community.
* During the project, communities were involved in field level steering
committees that included local representatives of the ministries of Finance;
Social Action; Women, Children and Family Affairs, and Health; the project's executing agency; women's leaders, leaders of youth clubs and
other local associations and nongovernmental organizations; and local
religious leaders. These committees helped with information exchange,
synchronization of activities, and building good interpersonal relations
and commitment.

Source: World Bank (2001b).

C. India: The Tamil Nadu Integrated Nutrition Project— attention to microlevel design and management

* *Recruitment criteria:* Outreach workers had to be from their local community. In addition, as much as possible, they were chosen from women
who were poor, but whose children were nevertheless well nourished.
Before they even began nutrition counseling, they were proof to the community that poverty need not be an impediment to good nutrition.

- *Work routines:* These were clearly defined on a daily, weekly, and monthly basis. Growth monitoring, for example, was conducted on the same three days every month, so women knew when to bring their children to the nutrition center. This cut down the number of home visits workers had to make to monitor children.
- *Supervision and training:* There was a field supervisor for every 10 community workers, and a senior supervisor for every 60–70 workers. The training system was innovative in that the senior supervisor was also the preservice and in-service trainer of the workers in her area. This meant training could be tailored to workers' individual needs and cut out the expense of maintaining a network of training institutions.
- *MIS:* Every month, data showing the proportion of children weighed and the number malnourished were posted on a chalkboard outside the nutrition center. This helped communities monitor progress. And every month, the data for all centers were analyzed by computer, and poor-performing centers were identified for special attention by supervisors—"management by exception."

Source: Heaver (2003a).

D. Honduras: The AIN-C program— attention to microlevel design and management

AIN-C (Atención Integral a la Niñez en la Comunidad—Integrated Attention to Childhood in the Community) aims to promote self-reliance. The focus is on helping families improve the care of children under age two with their own resources, based on research showing that 92 percent of families had adequate food resources and that the reasons for child malnutrition were largely behavioral. This is different from programs that assume the family cannot adequately provide for its children, and immediately offer food, coupons, or cash to parents with malnourished children.

AIN's field level management system has been carefully refined over a decade, and incorporates best practices from other community-based programs. Key features include:

Keeping it simple. Like the Tamil Nadu Integrated Nutrition Project (TINP), AIN focuses on child growth, rather than nutritional status. But unlike TINP, AIN's growth monitoring system does not rely on workers plotting each child's growth monthly on a graph. Instead, workers are given a table with figures showing how much weight a child of a given age (in years and months) should be putting on each month. They then have to make only a yes/no decision about whether the child's weight gain is adequate compared to the table. If not, workers discuss with the mother what is causing slow growth and agree on specific behavioral changes for improvement.

Workers have counseling cards, developed through a trials of improved practices (TIPs) formative research process, to help them tailor their advice to the family's particular situation. The card helps workers differentiate their advice by the child's age, adequacy or inadequacy of weight gain, illness status, and breastfeeding status. The card may suggest several areas for improvement, but the worker selects only one or two behaviors that the mother is willing to follow in the ensuing month. These could be as simple as nursing from both breasts at each feeding, or giving half of a tortilla to the child at two meals during each day. Next month, the mother gets feedback in the form of the child's weight gain, showing whether the behavior change made a difference.

Progress monitoring is done through an innovative 5-bar graph (see below for an example), which tracks five simple indicators in each village each month: the number of children under age two in the community, the number weighed that month, the number gaining adequate weight, the number with inadequate weight gain, and the number gaining inadequate weight for two or more months.

Community action. Once a quarter, the previous month's monitoring data (see below) are reported to the community at a meeting at which the community at large makes decisions and works collectively for the betterment of its children. Collective action is key because many problems causing poor child growth go beyond the power of a family to correct: contaminated water sources, garbage disposal, childcare, and poor health center outreach are all problems that families need to work together to fix.

Treatment as well as prevention. Another important intervention is the detection, assessment, and treatment of common childhood illnesses, especially diarrhea and pneumonia, in children under age five. Once the community workers have mastered the core AIN program for children under age two, focused primarily on home-based preventive actions, they are trained in AIN's illness and newborn modules (based on the Integrated Management of Childhood Illnesses [IMCI] approach), which focuses more on identifying danger signs, expedited referral, and some community-initiated treatment. They are also given timers to diagnose the rapid breathing that indicates pneumonia and an antibiotic to treat it.

AIN is being studied and adapted by other countries, such as Bolivia, El Salvador, Ghana, Guatemala, Nicaragua, Uganda, and Zambia.

Source: Griffiths and McGuire (2005).

5-bar graph as presented to the community to stimulate discussion of changes in child growth over time

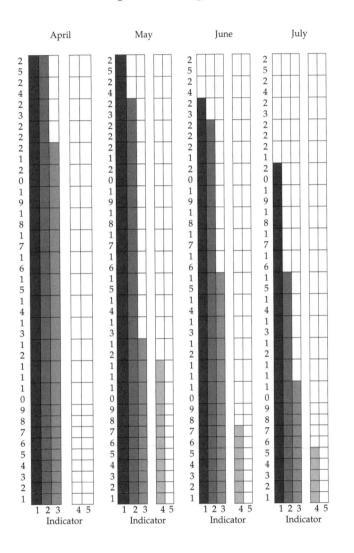

Indicators:
1. Number of children younger than 2 years listed in the register.
2. Number of children younger than 2 years who attended the weighing session this month.
3. Number of children younger than 2 years with adequate growth this month.
4. Number of children younger than 2 years with inadequate growth this month.
5. Number of children younger than 2 years with inadequate growth this month and last month.

E. Managing multisector programs: What not to do— experiences from World Bank–supported projects

- Rwanda's Food Security and Social Action Project initially put the finance ministry in charge of the project; it had no experience with program implementation and no presence in the field. Later in the project, inter-sectoral coordination was moved to the Ministry of Local Government, which handled it more successfully.
- In the Bangladesh Integrated Nutrition Project, the responsibility for multisectoral coordination was at too low a level to be effective. It was given to an Inter-Sectoral Nutrition Cell in the health ministry's project management unit, which had little influence over the other participating agencies—the Ministry of Agriculture and the Ministry of Fisheries and Livestock.
- No clear arrangements were made for managing nutrition as part of early childhood development (ECD) activities in Argentina's first World Bank–assisted Maternal and Child Health and Nutrition Project. The ECD centers had strong community support, but no institutional home in the government, not in the education ministry, whose focus was on schools, nor in the health ministry, which was more concerned with strengthening its own clinics than with nutrition outreach through preschool centers.

Source: World Bank Project Implementation Completion Reports.

F. Thailand: Incorporating nutrition into community development indicators—the village information system

Four government ministries (health, agriculture, education, and interior), led by the Ministry of Public Health, jointly developed the Basic Minimum Needs (BMN) system. It was piloted in Korat province in the northeast, and then picked up by the National Economic and Social Development Board, Thailand's planning ministry, and implemented nationwide.

There are 32 BMN indicators, divided into eight groups, as follows:

Adequate Food and Nutrition

1. Proper nutrition surveillance from birth to age five years and no moderate and severe protein-energy malnutrition (PEM).
2. School children receive adequate food for nutritional requirements.
3. Pregnant women receive adequate and proper food, and delivery of newborn babies with birthweight not less than 3,000 grams.

Proper Housing and Environment

4. The house will last at least five years.
5. Housing and the environment are hygienic and in order.
6. The household possesses a hygienic latrine.
7. Adequate clean drinking water is available all year round.

Adequate Basic Health and Education Services

8. Full vaccination with BCG, DPT, OPV, and measles vaccine for infants under one year of age.
9. Primary education for all children.
10. Immunization with BCG, DPT and typhoid vaccine for primary school children.
11. Literacy among citizens 14 to 50 years old.
12. Monthly education and information in health care, occupation, and other important areas for the family.
13. Adequate antenatal services.
14. Adequate delivery and postpartum services.

Security and Safety of Life and Properties

15. Security of people and properties.

Efficiency in Food Production by the Family

16. Growing alternative crops or soil production crops.
17. Utilization of fertilizers to increase yields.
18. Pest prevention and control in plants.
19. Prevention and control of animal diseases.
20. Use of proper genetic plants and animals.

Family Planning

21. Not more than two children per family and adequate family planning services.

People's Participation in Community Development

22. Each family is a member of self-help activities.
23. The village is involved in self-development activities.
24. Care of public properties.
25. Care and promotion of culture.

26. Preservation of natural resources.
27. People are active in voting.
28. The village committee is able to plan and implement projects.

Spiritual or Ethical Development

29. Being cooperative and helpful in the village.
30. Family members are involved in religious practices once per month.
31. Neither gambling nor addiction to alcohol or other drugs by family members.
32. Modest living and expenses.

Source: Heaver and Kachondam (2002).

G. Thailand: Sequenced partnership-building—making nutrition everybody's business

Building a constituency at the technical level

Thailand's three nutrition champions (two from the health sector and one from agriculture) built up a broader group of "friends of nutrition" across the government by sending key staff from the planning ministry and line agencies for overseas nutrition training together, and through follow-up seminars combining staff from different government departments.

Involving civil society: Mass communication

The nutrition champions enlisted the support of the private sector to finance a much-repeated television ad, showing children in the northeast of the country who were so poor that they were reduced to eating earth to fill their stomachs. There was a nationwide sense of shame that this could happen in Thailand.

Bringing key policy makers on board

They convinced senior managers in the finance and planning ministries that putting money into nutrition was an investment rather than a social welfare expenditure, since it would make Thailand more productive and competitive. The military government saw the advantages of a multisectoral rural development program for national stability and security as well as for economic development.

Widening the consensus

Once commitment had been built up in central government, seminars for provincial governors helped to bring regional governments into the partnership. In the villages, all government agencies were involved in advocacy for community development, raising public awareness and encouraging people to volunteer.

Appropriate management arrangements: High-level support and organizational incentives

A national nutrition committee, chaired by the deputy prime minister and with representatives from all concerned line agencies, helped raise the profile of nutrition. Though financial allocations are controlled by the planning ministry, each line agency is responsible for managing its part of the multisector program, and so each feels that nutrition is its business.

Source: Heaver and Kachondam (2002).

H. China: Building commitment is not just about communication—the iodine deficiency control program

This $152 million World Bank–supported project, rated highly satisfactory, introduced new technologies in 200 firms in 31 provinces. Success factors included:

- Commitment to salt iodization was built before the project began, through informal dialogue with local representatives of the United Nations Development Programme (UNDP), United Nations Children's Fund (UNICEF), United Nations Industrial Development Organization (UNIDO), and WHO, before the World Bank became involved; and by political leaders' involvement in international meetings facilitated by the Micronutrient Initiative (MI).
- There was a systematic plan to ensure that high level political commitment was disseminated to stakeholders at all levels. Government allied with civil society—for example, the All China Women's Federation—to run public awareness campaigns on the importance of iodization. In addition:
  - A strong, legislative framework requiring salt to be iodized, and a strong regulatory framework to ensure that it actually happened, were developed.

- A free-standing project for iodine was carved out of a much larger health sector loan: this helped focus attention on the issue.
- The salt industry was put in the driver's seat of the project, and its authority and responsibility helped ensure commitment to effective iodization.
- The environment was favorable: a national focus on industrial reform meant that industry saw the project as an opportunity to modernize through the project's capacity-building work in management, monitoring, packaging, marketing, and quality control. Hence industry and the health ministry had a common goal in successful project implementation.
- A carefully planned implementation management framework was defined, so all stakeholders knew what was expected of them and were monitored.
- Senior World Bank management expressed strong interest in the project and actively monitored its progress.
- Strong coordination between the development partners and regular informal technical assistance from local UN agencies helped sustain commitment.
- There was continuity of both country and World Bank project teams.

Source: World Bank (2001a).

Annex 4.2
Nutrition as part of health services

Child growth and development interventions center on health and nutrition:

1. Breastfeed exclusively for the first six months of infant's life.
2. Then feed freshly prepared, energy and nutrient rich complementary foods while continuing breastfeeding for two years.
3. Ensure adequate micronutrients through the diet or supplementation.
4. Continue feeding sick children, and offer them more fluids.
5. Ensure that every pregnant woman has adequate antenatal care.
6. Ensure that children get a full course of immunizations.
7. Ensure that children in malaria-endemic areas sleep under insecticide-treated bednets.
8. Give appropriate home treatment for infections, especially oral rehydration for diarrhea and drugs for malaria.
9. Recognize when sick children need professional care and seek it.
10. Follow health workers' advice about treatment, follow-up, and referral.
11. Dispose of feces safely, and wash hands afterwards and before touching food.
12. Promote mental and social development through talking, playing, and providing a stimulating environment.

Source: Hill, Kirkwood, and Edmond (2004).

The BASICS approach to incorporating nutrition into health services

The Basic Support for Institutionalizing Child Survival (BASICS) Projects are U.S. Agency for International Development (USAID) contracts to fight needless childhood deaths in the developing world (see www.basics.org). The current $100 million BASICS contract began in October 2004. It helps expand effective child health interventions, such as newborn health, vitamin A supplementation and other essential nutrition actions, immunization, pediatric AIDS, the treatment of diarrhea and pneumonia, and malaria control. It supports activities to increase the use of child health and nutrition interventions by families, communities, and health systems.

Essential Nutrition Actions (ENA)* is an approach, developed as part of the BASICS project, to expand the coverage of six proven nutrition interventions through actions at health facilities, in communities, and through communications channels:

• Exclusive breastfeeding for six months.
• Adequate complementary feeding from about age 6 months to 24 months, with continued breastfeeding.
• Appropriate nutritional care of sick and severely malnourished children.
• Adequate intake of vitamin A for women and children.
• Adequate intake of iron for women and children.
• Adequate intake of iodine by all members of the household.

There has been experience with implementing ENA at the community level in Benin, Ethiopia, Ghana, Madagascar, and Senegal. ENA is also being incorporated into the pre-service of doctors and other health professionals in the medical schools and paramedical training institutions of Ethiopia, Ghana, and Madagascar. The table below illustrates how different nutrition actions can be incorporated into the routine work of health personnel.

Essential nutrition actions in health services

When you see clients for	You should provide	The content should be
Prenatal care	Breastfeeding counseling	Breastfeeding immediately after delivery, the importance of colostrums and exclusive breastfeeding (EBF), solving problems that prevent establishing breastfeeding, and mother's diet.
	Iron/folate supplements and counseling	One daily tablet (60 mg iron) throughout pregnancy for 6 months (180 tablets), counseling on side effects and compliance, and when and how to get more tablets

Essential nutrition actions in health services *(continued)*

When you see clients for	*You should provide*	*The content should be*
Delivery and postpartum care	Breastfeeding assistance and counseling (all maternities should follow the "10 Steps for Baby Hospitals").	Immediate initiation of breastfeeding, check for position and attachment, management of common problems, duration of EBF up to about six months, dangers of giving water or liquids, and how to express breast milk.
	Vitamin A supplement for mothers	One dose of 200,000 IU administered to the mother after delivery (within the first eight weeks).
Postnatal checks	Exclusive breastfeeding check; reinforce good diet and rest for mothers.	Assess and counsel on problems, teach prevention of "insufficient milk," how to increase milk supply, manage problems, and mother's diet.
Immunizations	With tuberculosis vaccine (BCG) contact, check mother's vitamin A supplement.	Complete one dose of 200,000 IU for women within eight weeks after delivery (within six weeks if not breastfeeding).
	During National Immunization Days (NIDs) and community outreach for immunizations, check and complete children's vitamin A.	One dose of 100,000 IU for infants age 6–11 months; and one dose of 200,000 IU for children age 12–59 months, every 4–6 months.
	With OPV-3 and measles immunization, check infant's vitamin A.	One dose of 100,000 IU for infants age 6–11 months; and one dose of 200,000 IU for children age 12–59 months should be given every 4–6 months (for infants under age 6 months, use 50,000 IU per dose).

Essential nutrition actions in health services *(continued)*

When you see clients for	*You should provide*	*The content should be*
Well-baby visits	Assess and counsel on breastfeeding; assess and counsel on adequate complementary feeding (use locally adapted recommendations).	Counseling and support for EBF in the first 6 months, counseling and support for adequate complementary feeding from age 6–24 months, continuation of breastfeeding to age 24 months. Use iodized salt for all family meals.
	Check and complete vitamin A, iron, and antimalarial protocol.	See protocols above under immunizations, INNACG (1998).
Sick child visits	Screen, treat, and refer severe malnutrition, vitamin A deficiency, and anemia.	IMCI and WHO (1997) protocols for severe malnutrition, vitamin A deficiency, and anemia.
	Check and complete vitamin A protocol.	See protocols above under immunizations. Also provide vitamin A supplements for measles, diarrhea, and malnutrition according to WHO/UNICEF/IVACG.
	Assess and counsel on breastfeeding; assess and counsel on adequate complementary feeding (use locally adapted recommendations).	Increase breastfeeding while child is sick. Counsel and support EBF in the first 6 months; counsel and support for adequate complementary feeding for age 6–24 months, continuation of breastfeeding to age 24 months. Continued and recuperative feeding for sick children.

Source: Sanghvi and others (2003).
Note: * Acharya and others (2004).

Annex 5.1
Areas of focus in nutrition among development partners, by subject area

Types	Organizations	General malnutrition	Micronutrients	HIV and nutrition	Food policy/agriculture/rural development	Nutrition in maternal and child health/child feeding
UN agencies	UNICEF	X	X	X		X
	SCN*	X	X	X	X	X
	WFP		X	X		
	WHO**	X	X	X	X	X
	FAO			X	X	
Multilateral agencies	World Bank	X	X	X	X	X
	ADB	X	X		X	X
Bilateral agencies	DFID				X	
	SIDA				X	
	CIDA		X			
	USAID	X	X	X	X	X
	GTZ				X	X

	Organization						
	DANIDA						X
	NORAD						
	JICA					X	
	Dutch					X	
	Ireland AID	X			X		
Public/private partnerships	GAIN			X	X		
Private sector/NGOs	WABA			X			
	Manoff Group					X	X
	AED			X		X	
	HKI		X			X	
	MI		X				
	MOST		X				
	CARE			X		X	X
	La Leche League						
	FANTA		X			X	X
	BASICS		X	X			X
Research institutions	Harvest Plus			X		X	X
	IFPRI/CGIAR		X			X	X

Note: Tables 5.1 and 5.2 are indicative only and are based on a subjective review of Web sites and common knowledge about the focus of each organization.

*Functions primarily as a coordination body.

**Functions primarily as a technical body.

Annex 5.2
Areas of focus in nutrition among development partners, by technical area

Organizations		Commitment building			Capacity development			Mainstreaming nutrition into PRSCs, PRSPs and SWAps			Monitoring and evaluation			Research		
		G	N	SN	G	N	SN	G	N	SN	G	N	SN	T	A	O
UN agencies	UNICEF	X	X	X	X											X
	SCN	X	X													
	WFP	X			X											
	WHO	X			X						X					X
	FAO*	X				X					X					
Multilateral agencies	World Bank	X	X		X	X		X			X	X			X	
	ADB	X	X		X	X						X			X	X
Bilateral agencies	DFID*							X							X	
	SIDA															
	CIDA				X											
	USAID					X					X					

	Organization	G	N	SN	T	A	O
	GTZ	X					X
	DANIDA	X					
	NORAD			X			
	JICA	X					
	Ireland AID						
Public/private partnerships	GAIN***	X				X	
Private sector / NGOs	WABA**	X		X			
	Manoff Group			X			
	AED	X		X			
	HKI	X		X			X
	MI***	X		X		X	X
	MOST***	X		X		X	X
	CARE	X	X				
	La Leche League**	X					
	FANTA			X			X
	BASICS	X		X		X	X
Research institutions	Harvest Plus*	X				X	
	IFPRI/CGIAR	X				X	X

Note: G-Global; N-National; SN-Subnational;

T-Technological research; A-Applied research; O-Operational research.

* Focus primarily on food security.

** Focus primarily on infant feeding/breastfeeding.

*** Focus primarily on micronutrients.

Annex 5.3
Mandate and focus of development partners in nutrition

(Information for this annex has been extracted primarily from the Web sites of the relevant agencies/groups.)

Institutions	Mission statement/ mandate	Nutrition strategy
UN agencies		
WHO/ Department of Nutrition for Health and Development (NHD)	The importance of WHO's role in promoting nutrition is well elucidated. "Because of the fundamental role nutritional well-being plays in health and human development, and the world-wide magnitude of malnutrition-related mortality and morbidity, WHO has always included nutrition promotion, and the prevention and reduction of malnutrition, among its key health-promotion instruments."	• WHO shares responsibility with UNICEF in reporting on child mortality, maternal health, nutritional status, etc. • WHO, along with the Food and Agricultural Organization (FAO), convened International Conference on Nutrition, 1992. • Key documents include: **Turning the Tide of Malnutrition: Responding to the Challenge of the 21st Century; Nutrition for Health and Development: A global agenda for combating malnutrition, 2000.** • Consistent with nine goals and nine strategies of the World declaration and Plan of Action for Nutrition, NHD works through seven priority areas of action through a multisectoral framework. • The main objectives: 1. Capacity building for assessing and addressing nutrition-related problems; development of nutrition policies and programs. 2. Help develop scientific knowledge, methodologies, standards, strategies, etc., for detecting and preventing all forms of malnutrition deficiencies and excesses, including improvements in horticulture and farming systems.

Mandate and focus of development partners in nutrition (continued)

Institutions	Mission statement/ mandate	Nutrition strategy
WHO/NHD cont.		3. Promote sustainable health and nutrition benefits of targeted food and development projects. Works with World Food Program (WFP) to ensure effectiveness of food aid interventions. 4. Maintains global database for monitoring and evaluation (M&E) and reporting on world's major forms of malnutrition, effectiveness of programs, and achievement of targets at national, regional, and global levels. • The seven priority areas are: *PEM:* Management of severe malnutrition; spearheading a study to recalculate and overhaul existing growth curves: 1. *Micronutrients:* With partners, NHD provides technical tools, scientific standards, guidelines and methodologies to build up national programs, such as salt iodization programs; evaluates iodine deficiency disorders (IDD) programs in collaboration with UNICEF; maintains the global databank on IDD; promotes breastfeeding, supplementation, food fortification, and home gardens for eradicating vitamin A deficiencies; increases iron intake and infection control; and conducts research on vitamin A supplementation. 2. *Obesity:* Raising awareness; developing strategies that will make healthy choices easier to make; collaborating to calculate economic impact of obesity and to analyze the impact of globalization and rapid economic transition on nutrition.

Mandate and focus of development partners in nutrition (continued)

Institutions	Mission statement/ mandate	Nutrition strategy
WHO/NHD cont.		3. *Infant feeding:* • Promoting baby-friendly hospital initiative with UNICEF. • Intensifying technical support to improve complementary feeding practices. 4. *Emergencies:* Provision of manuals and guidelines on managing nutrition in emergencies; rapid nutrition assessments; promoting safe-feeding practices; and caring for the nutritionally vulnerable. 5. *Guiding food aid for development:* • WHO's Food Aid for Development (FAD) office assists elaboration of WFP's policies, guidelines, and country programs. • It assists WFP in identification, formulation, and evaluation of supplementary feeding programs. 6. *Developing effective food and nutrition polices and programs:* • WHO sees household food security as a basic human right. Undertaking a multicountry, multidisciplinary study since 1995 examining causal factors of malnutrition. • Other priority areas include developing global nutrition data banks and global network of collaborating centers in nutrition • Advisory group on Nutrition and HIV/AIDS.
UNICEF	Mandated to advocate for the protection of children's rights, to help meet their basic needs, and to	Nutrition strategy embodies their conceptual framework developed in 1990. Focus areas include: 1. *Micronutrients:* Works with governments in both donor and developing countries to develop innovative programs to deliver micronutrients

Mandate and focus of development partners in nutrition (continued)

Institutions	Mission statement/ mandate	Nutrition strategy
UNICEF, cont.	expand their opportunities to reach their full potential. Nutrition is one of the eight key program areas implied in the medium-term strategic framework. A new health and nutrition strategy is under development.	in foods or through health care services (salt iodization, folate, capsules and vitamin A supplementation) (DFID is a partner supplying capsules). Assists countries to formulate and use national recommendations on multi-micronutrients. • Not much focus on food-based strategies. 2. *Infant and child feeding:* • Promotion of EBF, timely introduction of complementary foods. • Also on the forefront of developing policy guidelines for infant feeding in HIV; capacity building of national institutions to develop their own guidelines and training, including training in counseling of mothers in infant feeding choices. • Immunization Plus as part of Child Health Weeks, including malaria components in some countries. 3. *Maternal nutrition/low birthweight:* Low-Birthweight Prevention Initiative is being piloted in 11 countries. The initiative includes the use of multiple micronutrient supplements for pregnant women. • Will complement UNICEF's Care for Women and Children Initiative, which focuses on women's education, workload, physical health and nutrition status, emotional well-being, reproductive health, and care during pregnancy and lactation. 4. *Growth Monitoring and Promotion (GMP):* • Working with WHO to develop new international growth references. Support for growth monitoring in more than 40 countries. • Expansion of therapeutic centers for severely malnourished children, especially in emergencies.

Mandate and focus of development partners in nutrition (continued)

Institutions	Mission statement/ mandate	Nutrition strategy
UNICEF, cont.		5. *Community-based programs:* • Strengthens local capacities to run such programs. • Triple A approach (assessment, analysis, action) for community mobilization. 6. *Nutrition information and surveillance systems:* • Supports generation of data on many key indicators of children's and women's well-being, including their nutrition status. • Supports updated data on selected nutrition indicators in the "childinfo" Web site. 7. *Emergencies: Most of the above in emergencies.* • National and regional nutrition surveillance to analyze the possible links between malnutrition and HIV/AIDS in Southern Africa.
WFP	As the food aid arm of the UN, WFP uses its food to: • Meet emergency needs. • Support economic and social development. "Works to put hunger at the center of the international agenda, promoting policies, strategies, and operations that directly benefit the poor and hungry."	*Strategic and Financial Plan 2002–5:* The goal for 2002–5 is: "Excellence in providing food assistance that enables all planned beneficiaries of WFP relief activities to survive and maintain healthy nutritional status, and enabling the social and economic development of at least 30 million hungry people every year." • Aligning future polices and operations with "Enabling Development." Policies and guidelines currently exist for procurement and for donors. • Development activities are envisioned to enable hungry poor to work toward sustainable food security, adequate nutrition, and economic development. • Combating micronutrient deficiencies: • Production and low-cost blended foods, including building national capacities (pilot in Ethiopia, India, Madagascar, North Korea, and Malawi). • Piloting standardization of premixed blended foods.

Mandate and focus of development partners in nutrition (*continued*)

Institutions	Mission statement/ mandate	Nutrition strategy
WFP, cont.		• Provision of fortified commodities—oil and blended food, especially in emergencies, high-energy biscuits, iodized salt, wheat, and maize flour fortified with vitamins and minerals. • Training staff and NGOs in nutrition issues. • Research on dietary diversity as an indicator of food security, and on ration composition quality in relation to nutrition outcomes. Project review committee screens all food interventions and examines quality and appropriateness. Supports research on the micronutrient impact of fortified biscuits derived from wheat. Supports research into effectiveness of blanket complementary food distribution for malnutrition prevention (Haiti). • Monitors the cost effectiveness of local purchases within country redistribution of foods. *Enabling Development (1999); Reaching mothers and children at critical times of their lives (1997):* • Supplementary feeding using blended foods. • School feeding (especially girls), as women's education could potentially reduce child malnutrition. • Improving livelihoods route to improving nutrition. • Acting early: Improving Vulnerability Analysis Mapping (VAM). **Emerging issues:** • Urban food insecurity and HIV. • *Urban food insecurity:* process of understanding the complex socioeconomic issues, informal safety nets, and how they respond to crisis. • *HIV:* policy statement (October 2002 draft).

Mandate and focus of development partners in nutrition (continued)

Institutions	Mission statement/ mandate	Nutrition strategy

UN Standing Committee on Nutrition (SCN)	The mandate of SCN is to:
	• Raise awareness of nutrition problems and mobilize commitment to solve them—at global, regional, and national levels.
	• Refine the direction, increase the scale, and strengthen the coherence and impact of actions against malnutrition worldwide.
	• Promote cooperation among UN agencies and partner organizations in support of national efforts to end malnutrition in this generation.
		Three main areas for action:
		1. Promote harmonized approaches among the UN agencies, and between the UN agencies and governmental and non-governmental partners, for greater overall impact on malnutrition.
		2. Review the UN system response to malnutrition overall, monitor resource allocation, and collate information on trends and achievements reported to specific UN bodies.
		3. Advocate and mobilize to raise awareness of nutrition issues at global, regional, and country levels and mobilize accelerated action against malnutrition.
		Ending Malnutrition by 2020: An Agenda for Change in the Millennium. Final Report to the ACC/SCN by the Commission on the Nutrition Challenges of the 21st Century, February 2000.
		• Proposes a new paradigm of nutrition, which incorporates the double burden of undernutrition and diet-related adult diseases.
		• Focus on preventable disorders in middle and old age.
		• Why have global plans of action such as International Conference on Nutrition (ICN) and World Food Summit (WFS) not achieved more?
		  • Lack of motivated actors to drive the nutrition agenda.
		  • Failure of health and agriculture sectors to combine forces for a coherent action. Lack of intersectoral approach highlighted.
		New agenda identifies four major tasks:
		1. Assessment of national policies and plans developed in response to SCN.
		2. Coordination of UN efforts.

Mandate and focus of development partners in nutrition *(continued)*

Institutions	Mission statement/ mandate	Nutrition strategy
SCN, cont.		3. New mechanism for developing national polices for diet and physical activity. The commission proposes National Nutrition Councils based on Norwegian and Thai experiences. 4. Acceptance of National Nutrition Councils to be the major focus for international support.
FAO/ Economic and Social Department/ Food and Nutrition Division (ESN)	Food and Nutrition Division aims to: • Raise awareness of the benefits of combating hunger and reducing malnutrition. • Assist countries in identifying people who are food-insecure and vulnerable to nutritional problems. • Promote food safety and prevent foodborne diseases. • Focus on consumer protection and fair practices in food trade.	ESN is responsible for: • Maintaining food and nutrition country profiles. • Stimulating and maintaining analysis of food composition data (INFOODS). • Nutrition assessments and monitoring, including FIVIMS, State of Food Insecurity in the World Reports, and FAO statistical databases on foods available for consumption. • Organizing consultations on nutrient requirements with other key partners. • Building the necessary program activities and support at the government and institutional levels to respond to identified needs, and thus reverse the situation; working on understanding urban nutrition, incorporating nutritional needs in NARS agenda. • Identify best practices, monitor impact on behavior, consumption, biochemistry, and function. • Initiatives to develop appropriate locally based complementary foods. • Provide fortification recommendations and technical assistance on food legislation, standards and food control, and quality assurance. In collaboration with WHO, provide standards and guidelines for labeling, nutrition and health claims, and nutritional quality.

Mandate and focus of development partners in nutrition (*continued*)

Institutions	Mission statement/ mandate	Nutrition strategy
FAO, cont.	• It has primary responsibility for coordinating FAO nutrition-related activities in follow-up to international meetings and agreements.	• Household Food Security and Community Nutrition Group, together with the Nutrition Information, Communication and Education Group (http://www. fao.org/es/ESN/nutrition/education_ en.stm), directs their activities toward developing and implementing effective community-centered programs: • Focus areas include food-based, community-centered approaches, including home gardens, food fortification, and preparing and planning for food emergencies. • Nutrition in HIV/AIDS. Developed guide, "Living well with HIV/AIDS." • Nutrition Information, Education, and Communication (IEC) Division's activities • Antihunger program: Reducing hunger through sustainable agriculture and rural development and wider access to food (FAO, Rome, 2002) (http://www.fao.org/DOCREP/004/Y715 1E/Y7151e00.HTM).

Multilateral agencies

World Bank/Health, Nutrition, and Population (HNP)	*Mission statement of HNP:* "Assist clients to improve health, nutrition, and population outcomes of poor people and protect people from the impoverishing effects of illness, malnutrition, and high fertility."	• Supports a multisectoral approach (including Poverty Reduction Strategy Papers [PRSPs], sectorwide approaches [SWAps]) to nutrition that targets the poor, especially young children and their mothers. • Focuses on community nutrition programs, food fortification programs, and food policy reforms. • Increasing focus on micronutrient deficiencies, the impact of nutrition on education and learning ability, and early child development projects. • The Bank's nutrition strategy is explicitly being framed in terms of accelerating progress towards achieving nutrition relevant MDGs.

Mandate and focus of development partners in nutrition
(continued)

Institutions	Mission statement/ mandate	Nutrition strategy

HNP, cont.		• Investing in capacity development within the World Bank and also at the national levels to enable nutrition partners to be at the negotiating table when the reforms, SWAps, and PRSPs are discussed.
		 • Continued advocacy on how nutrition actions can best be positioned within the new programming environment.
		 • Health Systems Development (HSD) group, under HNP, in the next two to three years will reorient its activities to focus on building the global knowledge base and institutional support needed to help countries accelerate progress toward achieving their MDG targets.
		 • Sector Strategy: Health, Nutrition, and Population, 1997. Key objectives stated include:
		   • Improve the health, nutrition, and population outcomes of the poor, and to protect the population from the impoverishing effects of illness, malnutrition and high fertility.
		   • Enhance the performance of health care systems by promoting equitable access to preventive and curative health, nutrition, and population services that are affordable, effective, well managed, of good quality, and responsive to clients.
		   • Secure sustainable health care financing by mobilizing adequate levels of resources, establishing broad-based risk pooling mechanisms, and maintaining effective control over public and private expenditure.
		 • Bank-supported programs in agriculture and rural development, water and sanitation, social protection, early child development, and maternal and child health can have significant impact on nutrition.

Mandate and focus of development partners in nutrition (continued)

Institutions	Mission statement/ mandate	Nutrition strategy
Asian Development Bank (ADB)	The Bank's overall approach to the health sector is to assist developing member country governments to ensure their citizens have broad access to basic preventive, promotive, and curative services that are efficacious, cost-effective, and affordable. From: ADB. 1999. Policy for the Health Sector. Manila.	Activities in the health sector will be guided by five strategic considerations outlined in the Policy for the Health Sector (1999): • The Bank will work to improve the health of the poor, women, children, and indigenous peoples by: (a) increasing its lending for the health sector and maintaining its current emphasis on primary health care (including reproductive health, family planning, and selected nutrition interventions); and (b) focusing on vulnerable groups with particular attention to women, and measuring the extent to which the poor, women, and indigenous peoples have access to health services. • The Bank will maintain a focus on achieving tangible, measurable results by: (a) further strengthening monitoring and evaluation of all health sector activities; (b) emphasizing interventions with strong evidence of effectiveness; (c) improving the quality of loans at entry; and (d) improving implementation of health sector activities. • The Bank will support the testing of innovative approaches and the rapid deployment of effective and affordable new technologies through: (a) financing pilot tests of new approaches to health care financing, organization, and management; and (b) helping support the deployment of new technologies, particularly new vaccines. • The Bank will play a significant role in health sector reform by encouraging developing member country (DMC) governments to take an appropriate and activist role in the health sector. This will involve engaging in policy dialogue to encourage the DMCs to: (a) increase their budgetary allocations for primary health care; (b) diversify their sources of health care financing; (c) collaborate more extensively with the private sector; and

Mandate and focus of development partners in nutrition (*continued*)

Institutions	Mission statement/ mandate	Nutrition strategy
ADB, cont.		(d) increase support for public goods such as research, health education, and regulation. • The Bank will increase the efficiency of its health sector investments by: (a) helping to strengthen management capacity of the public sector in the DMCs; (b) improving its economic and sector work and strengthening linkages with other sectors; and (c) further strengthening its collaboration with partner institutions operating in the health sector. A review of this policy is planned for 2005/2006, at which time it is anticipated nutrition and population considerations will be more explicitly considered and integrated into ADB's policy for the sector.

Bilaterals

Norway— Ministry of Foreign Affairs		Action Plan for Combating Poverty in the south toward 2015, March 2002: • Increase in development assistance to 1 percent of gross national income (GNI) by 2005. • Mentions education and health, but not nutrition.
NORAD Institutional set-up for nutrition not clear http://www. norad.no/	• NORAD aims to achieve lasting improvements in political, economic, and social conditions for the entire population within the limits imposed by the natural	"Nutritional considerations in Norwegian development cooperation" argues that NORAD should explicitly incorporate nutritional considerations in its plan for 2000-5. • Recommends supporting partner countries' national plan of action for food and nutrition in formulation and implementation. • Building or strengthening institutions • Supporting nutrition surveillance systems. (*Not clear if these recommendations have been implemented.*)

Mandate and focus of development partners in nutrition (*continued*)

Institutions	Mission statement/ mandate	Nutrition strategy
NORAD, cont.	environment and the natural resource base. • Has links to health/education and HIV, but not nutrition. Nutrition not even overtly mentioned.	Other key documents include: • Focus on NORAD: Statement to the starting on development cooperation policy 2002: Report on NORAD in 2002 (expands on the Action Plan). • Annual Report 2001—NORAD: Emphasizes that health and education are the most important areas of focus.
Denmark/ Danish International Development Agency (DANIDA)	• Danish assistance will in the future concentrate on its original main objective: promoting sustainable development through poverty-oriented economic growth. • A critical review conducted in 2002. Results will appear in appropriation bill of 2003.	• No clear nutrition strategy mentioned. • But "to help poor by investing in education and health" is the primary goal. • More focus on women.
Japan/ Japanese International Co-operation Agency (JICA)	Technical assistance aimed to transfer technology and knowledge that can serve the socioeconomic development of the developing countries.	• Nutrition per se not prominent. • Priority areas are dependent on regional and country level issues. Therefore, JICA's priorities in South America are very different from Africa. • Food security, agriculture development, and health care are priority issues in Africa. In South America,

Mandate and focus of development partners in nutrition (*continued*)

Institutions	Mission statement/ mandate	Nutrition strategy

JICA, cont.
 	
No institutional set-up for nutrition apparent
	http://www.jica.go. jp/english	issues include strengthening international competitiveness, environment-friendly agriculture, etc.
		• Global issues of concern include:
		  • Poverty, gender, environment, education, and health.
		  • Population and AIDS.
		  • Trade and peace building.
		  • Disability.

Canada/ Canadian International Development Agency (CIDA)/ Health and Nutrition	• "CIDA supports sustainable development activities in order to reduce poverty and to contribute to a more secure, equitable, and prosperous world." • Health and Nutrition: "Canada is active in promoting health and nutrition in developing countries and countries in transition, focusing on the poorest and most marginalized people—who are most often women and children."	• "Canada will commit 25 percent of its ODA to basic human needs as a means of enhancing its focus on addressing the security of the individual." • Under the priority area of "Basic human needs," CIDA supports health and nutrition. • Contributed to the creation of Micronutrient Initiative (MI). *Extract from CIDA's Action Plan on Health and Nutrition, 2001:* Guidelines through 2005: • Contribute to reduction in poverty by investing in health, nutrition, and water. • Rights-based approach, gender analysis. • Integrated and targeted nutrition programs: protecting women's nutrition, improving child feeding practices. • Vitamin A supplementation and salt iodization. • Food security: food-based strategies, emphasizes the need to develop new ways of examining impacts. • Has research and capacity development program for tropical diseases and reproductive health, but not nutrition.

Mandate and focus of development partners in nutrition (continued)

Institutions	Mission statement/ mandate	Nutrition strategy
Sweden/ Swedish International Development Agency (SIDA) Health and education are under the Department for Democracy and Social Development (DESO). There seems to be no house for nutrition.	The overall goal of Swedish development cooperation is to raise the standard of living of poor people in the world. The Swedish Parliament has adopted the following six specific objectives to achieve this overall goal: • Economic growth. • Economic and political independence. • Economic and social equality. • Democratic development in society. • The long-term sustainable use of natural resources and protection of the environment. • Equality between men and women.	Health Sector policy states that SIDA supports research, including malnutrition: • Emphasizes health sector development through bilateral and multilateral cooperation. • Malnutrition is mentioned as "other sectors" that could affect health. • SIDA's Poverty Programme 1996: Food security is one of the priority areas under the Department of Natural Resources and Environment. No elaboration provided. Key documents include: • SIDA Looks Forward—SIDA's Programme for Global Development (not available on line). • Policy for development cooperation: Health sector, 1997. • Perspectives on poverty, 2002 (fleeting mention of nutrition).
Germany/ German Agency for Technical Assistance (GTZ)		**GTZ:** Agriculture and agriculture research are priority areas. • The only publication on nutrition listed on the Web is on certification of organic foods.

Mandate and focus of development partners in nutrition (*continued*)

Institutions	Mission statement/ mandate	Nutrition strategy
Ireland Aid	The Government is committed, through its *Action Programme for the Millennium*, to reaching the target for development aid of 0.45 percent of gross national product (GNP) by the year 2002. http://www. irlgov.ie/iveagh/ irishaid/overview /default.htm	• Programs and projects to meet the basic needs include food security, health care, education, and clean water supplies. Report of the Ireland Aid review committee, February 2002 http://www.irlgov.ie/iveagh/irishaid/ irlaidreview.pdf: • It endorses its food security program. • No nutrition-specific strategy. Reaching the UN Target—A millennium decision for Ireland, Ireland Aid, 2000 http://www.irlgov.ie/iveagh/irishaid/ 2000report/IrelandAid.pdf

USAID	USAID places the highest priority on alleviating undernutrition and is focused on improving nutrition through sectoral programs in agriculture, health, food aid, population, and education as well as direct nutrition programs.	USAID'S strategy incorporates nutrition through its development assistance program by:
		 • Identifying projects based on nutrition and food consumption problems.
		 • Including nutrition as a factor in project design in:
		   • Agriculture projects.
		   • In health through primary health care.
		   • In food aid through targeting appropriate rations to at-risk groups.
		   • In population by complementing family planning services.
		   • In education through promotion of nutrition education in schools, training community health workers, providing advanced training for professionals.
		 • Targeting sectoral projects at individuals/households who are at risk to developing nutrition problems.
		 • Monitoring and evaluating nutrition impacts of projects.

Mandate and focus of development partners in nutrition (*continued*)

Institutions	Mission statement/ mandate	Nutrition strategy

USAID, cont.		• Complementing sectoral projects with nutrition projects.
		• Utilizing the private sector in food programs where feasible.
		• Encouraging the development of national policies.
		• Coordinating with less developed country (LDC) governments/donors to reach nutrition goals.
		• USAID has also developed a strategy to provide food and nutrition assistance in HIV/AIDS programs. Country programs include:
		  • **Rwanda:** USAID provides assistance to NGOs to provide food to approximately 29,000 children affected by HIV/AIDS as part of a comprehensive package of services.
		  • **Uganda:** USAID has a five-year, $30 million program, which is the largest of its kind in the world. The program targets approximately 60,000 individuals who have HIV/AIDS or live in households where providing HIV/AIDS care is undermining the ability to meet food and nutrition needs. The target population receives intensive nutrition education in addition to food aid. The program involves communities in food distribution to raise awareness, reduce stigma, and mobilize community involvement in HIV/AIDS activities.

U.K. Department for International Development (DFID)		DFID's strategy for achieving the MDG target of reducing hunger by 2015: • Promote a shared analysis of the causes of hunger and malnutrition and of progress towards the hunger MDG.

Mandate and focus of development partners in nutrition (continued)

Institutions	Mission statement/ mandate	Nutrition strategy
DFID, cont.		• Better integration of food security into poverty reduction efforts. • Promote the development of human capital. • Promote trade reforms that strengthen the food security of poor. • Better response to drought, conflict, and emergencies. • Better systems to identify who is hungry, where, and why. No explicit nutrition strategy. Proposed global nutrition priorities for DFID based on existing gaps (International Food Policy Research Institute [IFPRI] study, 2003): • Embed nutrition components within development actions. • Manage and generate practical knowledge at the intersection of livelihoods, the life-course, and lifestyles. • Develop capacity to integrate nutrition within sector initiatives. • Use and develop nutrition indicators to measure progress of nonnutrition activities • Highlight the key role of nutrition as both a driver of development and a nonexclusive investment opportunity.
Private Sector/NGOs		
Academy for Educational Development (AED) (Funding mainly from USAID and other partners)	AED helps communities secure stable food sources and improve their overall health and well-being.	AED is involved in several large projects, mostly funded by USAID, which outline its strategy for addressing the different aspects of nutrition: • **CHANGE PROJECT**—develops tools and strategies to facilitate individual and social behavior change relevant to child health, maternal health, infectious disease, and HIV/AIDS. A major focus is improving individual and household behaviors.

Mandate and focus of development partners in nutrition (continued)

Institutions	Mission statement/ mandate	Nutrition strategy
AED, cont.	With programs addressing issues such as breastfeeding, malnutrition, and food security, AED helps foster healthy communities around the world. AED is a leader in applying behavior change and social marketing methodologies to public health nutrition problems, particularly in breastfeeding, infant feeding, feeding of infants born to HIV-positive mothers, and micronutrient deficiencies. Over the last five years, AED has built up one of the largest concentrations of public health nutrition experts outside academia.	• **Ethiopia Child Survival and Systems Strengthening Project (ESHE)**—Focus of the project is to increase the survival rates of young children in Ethiopia through improved vaccination and nutritional supplementation. The program provides vitamin A, iron, and folate supplementation coverage for women and children and promotes exclusive breastfeeding for infants and continued breastfeeding to at least 24 months of age. • **Food and Nutrition Technical Assistance Project (FANTA)**—Supports integrated food security and nutrition programming. Helps integrate nutrition into the strategic planning process; provides analyses for food security and nutrition policy development, and shares information and knowledge with partners. • **LINKAGES**—This program focuses on increasing breastfeeding and related practices to improve maternal and reproductive health through technical assistance and training. • **Preventing Type II Diabetes (STOPP-T2D)** (funded by George Washington University)—This initiative is to design a social marketing strategy and communications program for middle schools in the United States to promote physical activity and healthy food choices. • **PROFILES** (multiple funders)—Engages national leaders in policy dialogue and public health nutrition. It has been credited with raising awareness about nutrition, building consensus, building capacity, and developing leadership skills of nutrition advocates.

Mandate and focus of development partners in nutrition (continued)

Institutions	Mission statement/ mandate	Nutrition strategy

AED, cont.	Areas of focus include policy analysis and advocacy, evaluation and monitoring, and comprehensive planning for food security.	• **Support for Analysis and Research in Africa (SARA)**—Provides assistance to African institutions to develop and promote policies to increase sustainability, quality, efficiency, and equity of a variety of health services, including nutrition.
		• **Useful tools and publications:**
		  • Breastfeeding and maternal nutrition: Frequently asked questions.
		  • Child health counseling cards, Dominican Republic.
		  • Community heath worker incentives and disincentives: How they affect motivation, retention and sustainability.
		  • Food and nutrition implications of ART in resource limited settings.
		  • HIV/AIDS Mitigation: Using what we already know.
		  • Quantifying the benefits of breastfeeding: A summary of the evidence.

Hellen Keller International (HKI)	Provide technical assistance, training, and M&E for homestead food production (gardening, fisheries, poultry, and animal husbandry).	• Research and Development: Development of dietary assessment methods; testing plant varieties and gardening methods; and developing and testing postflood gardening rehabilitation practices. Compliance with international code of breastfeeding. • Provide advice to agriculture ministries within countries to think about production of nongrain foods and appreciate the importance of food for better health. • Provide technical assistance and training to support ongoing programs with local partners in six countries in Africa and Asia. • Conduct surveillance and program monitoring to monitor anemia and iron deficiency, evaluate program coverage and the impact of homestead food production on nutrition status, household income, food consumption, and women's empowerment.

Mandate and focus of development partners in nutrition (continued)

Institutions	Mission statement/mandate	Nutrition strategy
HKI, cont.		• Conduct food surveys, including FRATs, to determine food patterns for fortification and the impact of iron-fortified candy. • Provide assistance to countries to develop guidelines, training, and materials to implement new policies on vitamin A supplementation for children postpartum and sick children. • Conduct operational research on anemia programs for school-age children and young infants and help develop national surveys to identify iron deficiency and the impact of interventions on anemia. • Integrate malaria and vitamin A in program interventions. • Monitor breastfeeding practices and evaluate program impact,
MI	The Micronutrient Initiative (MI) is a not-for-profit organization specializing in addressing micronutrient malnutrition. MI is governed by an international Board of Directors. MI supports and promotes food fortification and supplementation programs in Asia, Africa, and Latin America and	• Support for the Fresh Food Initiative (FFI), planning and implementation of national food fortification programs for iron, folic acid, and other nutrients, and technical guidelines. • Research and development: efficacy and effectiveness studies. Promote use of red palm oil by households and school feeding programs in West Africa; promote cultivation and use of orange-fleshed sweet potatoes in Southern Africa; efficacy of carotene-rich sweet potatoes in improving vitamin A staples; efficacy of double-fortified salt; impact of iron supplements on school performance. • Procure premix and equipment. • Conduct national and subnational impact evaluations. • Conduct vitamin A stability studies. • Provide program planning/implementation and technical assistance to governments and oil refining in core countries.

Mandate and focus of development partners in nutrition (*continued*)

Institutions	Mission statement/ mandate	Nutrition strategy
	provides technical and operational support in those countries where micronutrient malnutrition is most prevalent. MI carries out its work in partnership with other international agencies, governments, and industry.	• Pilot and scale up programs for production and distribution of complementary foods, as well as conduct research on the efficacy/ effectiveness of complementary foods. • Procure vitamin A capsules and support program implementation; design oral dropper technology; and develop field methods for biochemical assessment. • Promote and conduct impact studies on the effect of multiple micronutrient supplements for special feeding programs. • Provide expert training workshops and capacity building for understanding how to develop effective fortification programs. • Provide technical guidelines for flour fortification.

Private sector

Manoff Group	The Manoff Group provides assistance in communications and behavior-centered planning, management, and evaluations for health, nutrition, and population projects.	The Manoff Group addresses nutrition through a variety of programmatic approaches. • Strategic program design. • Consultative research: Trials on improved practices (TIPs) is the core method for the consultative research process. TIPs offers: • In-depth understanding of child feeding practices. • Adaptation of feeding recommendations to specific situations. • Understanding the motivations and constraints to change behavior. • Flexibility. • Quick and inexpensive field research. • A bridge between the nutrition program and the family and community. • Training in nutrition counseling.

Mandate and focus of development partners in nutrition (*continued*)

Institutions	Mission statement/ mandate	Nutrition strategy

Manoff Group, cont.		• Community mobilization: The Manoff Group has a variety of approaches, including community-based growth promotion model, community surveillance, and behavior change approach.
		• Product marketing: This is driven by a behavior change strategy based on formative, consultative research. Examples of products that Manoff Group projects have promoted are:
		  • Iron tablets in Indonesia, Pakistan, India, and Bolivia, among other countries.
		  • Vitamin A capsules in Thailand, Indonesia, and El Salvador, among other countries.
		  • Vitamin A–fortified sugar in Zambia, Bolivia, and El Salvador.
		  • Iron-fortified wheat products in Nicaragua.
		• Country program experience includes:
		  • Communicating importance of breastfeeding to families in Pakistan and Indonesia.
		  • Identification of/education on nutritious weaning foods in El Salvador, India, and Zambia.
		  • Community counseling on importance of nutrition for growth in Honduras and the Dominican Republic, among other countries.
		  • Micronutrient supplementation and nutrition education programs for school children in Egypt and Indonesia.
		  • Young child feeding in El Salvador, India, and Guatemala.
		• Manoff Group has produced useful resources for general health and nutrition communication, micronutrient malnutrition, maternal health, and environmental health.

Mandate and focus of development partners in nutrition (continued)

Institutions	Mission statement/ mandate	Nutrition strategy
Global Alliance for Improving Nutrition (GAIN)	GAIN's mandate is to forge an alliance of public, private, and civil society partners committed to eliminating vitamin and mineral deficiencies globally. GAIN has adopted the goals for country level operations from the United Nations General Assembly Special Session on Children in May 2002 to: • Achieve sustainable elimination of vitamin A deficiency by 2010. • Reduce anemia prevalence, including iron deficiency, by one-third by 2010. • Eliminate IDD by 2005. • Accelerate progress toward reduction of other vitamin and mineral deficiencies through dietary diversification,	GAIN will combine the strengths of public and private sector organizations to: • Mobilize private industry, international donors, and foundations in support of food fortification initiatives in low-income countries. • Tap the expertise and resources of the corporate sector in technology transfer, business development, trade, and marketing. • Work with the UN and other multilateral agencies to set international standards and establish systems for quality assurance and control. • Utilize public sector capabilities to address legislative and regulatory barriers to food fortification. • Develop a broader role for NGOs and civic organizations in food fortification. • Link food fortification efforts with other essential interventions, such as micronutrient supplementation and dietary diversification. N.B.: Fortification of staple foods and condiments is determined by country situation and not by GAIN. *Research and development:* • GAIN will prioritize research needs (global and regional) as well as capacity development. • GAIN follows a code of fortification and is developing a global advisory group on fortification within the context of the already existing WHO IMAGE. • Elevate nutrition on national agendas and further the MDGs.

Mandate and focus of development partners in nutrition
(continued)

Institutions	Mission statement/ mandate	Nutrition strategy
GAIN, cont.	food fortification, biofortification, and supplementation.	• Provide support to the National Food Authority (NFA) building partnerships.

Research Institutions

| IFPRI | • IFPRI's mission is to provide policy solutions that cut hunger and malnutrition. This mission flows from the CGIAR mission: "To achieve sustainable food security and reduce poverty in developing countries through scientific research and research-related activities in the fields of agriculture, livestock, forestry, fisheries, policy, and natural resources management." Two key premises underlie IFPRI's mission. First, sound and appropriate | IFPRI uses four sets of criteria to determine its priorities as part of its nutrition strategy: 1. The work program must conform to IFPRI's mission to provide policy solutions that reduce hunger and malnutrition. 2. Research and outreach should address emerging issues that most directly affect food security, nutrition, and poverty. 3. Research, capacity-strengthening, and policy-communications activities should be based on IFPRI's dynamic comparative advantage to produce results applicable to many countries—that is, international public goods. 4. Stakeholders and partners should be consulted to identify food policy research that all parties believe will help develop policies to reduce hunger and malnutrition. These criteria work as a decision tree: Research and outreach activities must meet all four criteria in order to be included on IFPRI's agenda.

IFPRI places a high priority on activities that benefit the greatest number of poor people in greatest need in the developing world. In carrying out its activities, IFPRI seeks to focus on vulnerable groups, as influenced by caste, class, religion, ethnicity, and gender. |

Mandate and focus of development partners in nutrition (continued)

Institutions	Mission statement/ mandate	Nutrition strategy
IFPRI, cont.	local, national, and international public policies are essential to achieving sustainable food security and nutritional improvement. Second, research and the dissemination of its results are critical inputs into the process of raising the quality of the debate and formulating sound and appropriate food policies. IFPRI's mission entails a strong emphasis on research priorities and qualities that facilitate change.	IFPRI is also committed to providing international food policy knowledge as a global public good; that is, it provides knowledge relevant to decision makers both inside and outside the countries where research is undertaken. New knowledge on how to improve the food security of low-income people in developing countries is expected to result in large social benefits, but in most instances the private sector is unlikely to carry out research to generate such knowledge. IFPRI views public organizations and the private sector in food systems both as objects of study and as partners. Given the large body of national and international food policy research, IFPRI's added value derives from its own cutting-edge research linked with academic excellence in other institutions, such as other Consultative Group on International Agricultural Research (CGIAR) centers, universities, and other research institutes in the South and North, and from its application of this knowledge to national and international food policy problems.
HarvestPlus	Biofortification is a strategy of getting plants to fortify their seeds/roots through plant breeding. An interdisciplinary global alliance of research institutions and implementing	• Research and development is the main focus of HarvestPlus. • Conducts research on food and agricultural policies that impact the dietary quality of the poor; conducts cost benefit analyses of alternative interventions and efficacy trials. • Develops social marketing messages such as encouraging consumers to switch from white to consumption of yellow/orange varieties in breeding

Mandate and focus of development partners in nutrition (*continued*)

Institutions	Mission statement/ mandate	Nutrition strategy
HarvestPlus, cont.	agencies has been assembled to develop bio-fortified vari-eties and to dis-seminate them to farmers in developing countries. HarvestPlus is the name of this global program.	vitamin A carotenoids; develops messages to promote food and agricultural policies that enhance dietary quality. • Collaborates with government extension agencies, NGOs, and private sector to disseminate biofortified varieties by working through established seed markets and developing new seed markets as necessary.

Annex 5.4
Deciding how to invest in nutrition: A framework for making policy choices

Deciding how best to improve nutrition can be a controversial process because:

- Many different interventions can have an effect on nutrition.
- At least 10 variables need to be taken into account in deciding what to do.
- Needs, priorities, and constraints vary between countries, between regions and population groups within countries, and over time, so generalizing is impossible.
- People see different priorities for action, depending on their understanding about what causes malnutrition and their knowledge about the range of possible interventions.
- There are often vested interests in expanding one type of program rather than another.

The biggest impact on malnutrition comes from multisectoral programs that include most of the menu of nutrition interventions set out in table 3.1 of the main volume of this report. But for various reasons—because they lack the commitment, or the funds, or the managerial capacity—most countries where malnutrition is serious cannot expect to implement a broad, multisectoral nutrition program on a national scale, at least in the short and medium term. The issue is how such countries, which cannot do everything, should decide what to do as a priority.

Here are six sets of questions that provide a framework for decision making. While it makes sense to consider them initially in the order presented, the decision-making process needs to be iterative, since the answers to some later questions may require reconsideration of earlier questions. Who addresses these questions is as important as how they are addressed. The more stakeholders that are involved in the policy choice process, the more chaotic and difficult it is likely to be. On the other hand, the more stakeholders that have been involved and hence understand the rationale for policy decisions, the greater the likelihood of commitment to implementing the chosen policies.

Question 1: How does the environment constrain what can be done, and what opportunities does it offer?

The different nutrition options need to be considered in the context of the political, cultural, institutional, and financial environment. A situation analysis is therefore the first step in the policy choice process, focusing on both constraints and opportunities.

Constraints

Questions to ask include:

- Is government commitment to poverty reduction, to human development, and to improving nutrition real, or mainly rhetoric?
- Are politicians committed to nutrition programs (some food subsidy programs, school feeding) that bring political benefits, but have little impact on nutrition?
- How far do public expenditure constraints limit what new initiatives can be taken?
- How far do managerial constraints limit what new initiatives can be taken?
- Do governance problems hamper the implementation of social sector programs?
- What are the limitations of the available nutrition data and the capacity to analyze it?

Opportunities

Questions to ask include:

- What policies and programs do politicians favor, and how might investing in nutrition further their goals?
- What cultural values might support increased attention to nutrition, and what community organizations or mutual help traditions might facilitate program implementation?
- What small-scale nutrition interventions exist that might be made more cost-effective and scaled up?
- What existing nutrition-related programs—in health, agriculture, social protection, and water and sanitation—have institutional capacity that can be built on?
- What institutional capacity is there outside government—NGOs, social research institutes, commercial consultants?

Question 2: What makes the most technical and economic sense?

The variables to be taken into account here are epidemiology and cost-effectiveness.

Epidemiology

The type of malnutrition problem, its extent and seriousness, what causes it, and who suffers from it (age groups, sex, and geographical location) all need to be reviewed. Countries vary greatly in their epidemiological needs:

- In many middle and high-income countries, overnutrition is the main manifestation of malnutrition, and interventions in nutrition education and food policy are the corresponding priorities.
- Micronutrient malnutrition is a problem in more than 55 countries, both low and middle income. Food fortification is a solution for the population at large, but supplementation is needed for high-risk groups—for example, for anemic pregnant women who need more iron than they can absorb just from fortified foods.
- Protein-energy malnutrition (PEM) is a problem in more than 60 countries. Here, looking at what causes it is crucial. The most common cause of PEM is parents' poor child feeding and caring practices, and the corresponding solution is growth monitoring and education about breastfeeding and weaning, as well as better diets for pregnant and lactating women. But if disease is an important cause of malnutrition, then health, water, or sanitation interventions can be as important; and if food security is a problem, then indirect interventions against malnutrition should be considered (see below). UNICEF's food-health-care framework for understanding the causes of malnutrition is useful here (UNICEF 1990).
- Both micronutrient malnutrition and PEM are a problem in more than 50 countries.

Cost-effectiveness

The direct interventions against malnutrition are all cost-effective. But relative cost-effectiveness varies between interventions and in different country circumstances, for example:

- While both PEM and micronutrient interventions are cost-effective ways to reduce malnutrition, micronutrient interventions are relatively more cost-effective (Lomborg 2004) because they cost less per client and are easily added to existing health programs.

- If a country has already invested in one type of program, it is often more cost-effective to improve or expand that, rather than create a new, different type of program because extra investment at the margin of an existing program to remove bottlenecks to performance usually has a very high payoff.

Cost-effectiveness and epidemiological considerations need to be balanced. Globally, growth promotion programs focusing on improving caring practices have been neglected because there have been lobbies for investing in health and agriculture, but not in care. Yet poor caring practices are probably the biggest worldwide cause of PEM. So countries need to be careful about investing only in cheap micronutrient programs or in expanding food security programs because they are already in place if they have a caring practice problem that is not being systematically addressed.

Question 3: What will actually work on the ground?

The key variables here are commitment, capacity, and affordability.

Commitment

Nutrition programs get off the ground, and get sustained, only if key politicians, officials, and local communities are committed to them. So investment decisions should not be taken only on the basis of what is technically and economically rational, but also on the basis of what is politically rational. For example, investments in children are often politically popular. So tackling malnutrition through child development programs can make political sense, as well as reaping benefits from the synergy between improving health, nutrition, and early stimulation simultaneously. Approaches for assessing commitment are suggested in Heaver (2005b).

Capacity

Countries' limited technical capacity often constrains their ability to design nutrition programs, and limited management capacity often constrains their ability to expand programs, ensures their quality, and makes service providers accountable for results. When capacity is limited, it makes sense to start with nutrition interventions that build on existing capacity. It is usually possible to build on existing health system capacity: one example is incorporating vitamin A supplementation into outreach services for immunization; another is incorporating nutrition into health clinic services using the IMCI approach. Food fortification uses the existing capacity of private sector food manufacturers and distributors. And several governments have successfully used existing NGO capacity to deliver growth promotion outreach services.

Affordability

Sometimes nutrition interventions can have a high impact and be highly cost-effective without being affordable at scale. Small-scale, donor-financed projects frequently develop effective but expensive interventions without considering whether they can be scaled up. So it is essential for governments and development partners to get together and decide to test out in projects only things that have a chance of going to scale. Examples of interventions that usually are affordable at scale because they are relatively cheap are vitamin A and iodine supplementation, food fortification, and IMCI.

Question 4: What is the right balance between direct and indirect interventions?

The direct interventions are usually the most cost-effective way to improve nutrition. A list of what are commonly defined as the direct (short route) interventions is given in table 3.1 of the main volume of this report.

There is some confusion about where food stands as an intervention. Traditionally, food security interventions are classified as indirect, because, while they improve *household* food security, they may not directly affect the nutritional status of *at-risk family members*—infants, for example. But it seems inappropriate to classify food as an indirect intervention where it does directly improve nutritional status, as with, for example:

- Food supplements targeted on growth-faltering children under age three in the TINP (Heaver 2003a). These both directly improved their nutrition and taught mothers about the nutritional benefits of feeding small amounts of extra food.
- Food supplementation targeted on low-BMI pregnant women in Bangladesh (Pelletier, Shekar, and Du forthcoming), which substantially improved their nutritional status.
- Food aid geographically targeted on families in drought-affected areas of Ethiopia, which likewise had direct nutritional benefits (Yamano, Alderman, and Christiaensen 2004). Food aid for families uprooted by conflict, or without able-bodied adults due to war or AIDS, is another example.

- Food-for-work schemes that are targeted seasonally so families can maintain their food consumption during the preharvest lean season, or when harvests fail.

Targeted food supplementation can therefore be direct intervention. A useful review of advantages and disadvantages of different food-based safety nets can be found in Rogers, Lorge, and Coates (2002).

The indirect interventions are usually a second order investment priority for improving nutrition. But they can be first order priorities under certain country circumstances. For example:

- Immunization is a priority wherever coverage is low, since the common infectious diseases cause children's growth to falter.
- Oral rehydration is a priority wherever diarrhea is a leading cause of malnutrition, and water supply and sanitation programs can also be effective in reducing diarrhea (Fewtrell and Colford 2004).
- Treatment for malaria and intestinal parasites may be a high priority wherever high parasite loads weaken children's ability to absorb nutrients.

Otherwise, the relative cost-effectiveness of the indirect interventions seldom justifies financing them in preference to direct interventions on purely nutritional grounds. For example, stimulating economic growth improves nutrition, but it takes so long to change nutritional status that it is not a priority nutrition intervention—although, of course, economic growth is needed to reduce income poverty, and to finance the taxes that pay for direct nutrition programs. But governments finance many indirect interventions anyway, with the aim of reducing income poverty. Where such interventions are already being financed, steps can often be taken to design them so they have an impact on nutrition as well as incomes. For example:

- By targeting livelihood creation programs on families suffering from malnutrition, as with the poultry-rearing activities in Bangladesh's National Nutrition Program.
- By combining microcredit/income generation programs with nutrition education, which increases the likelihood of some of the extra income being spent on improving nutrition.
- By coordinating the implementation of water and sanitation and health and nutrition programs so as to maximize their synergy, as in Honduras's Nutrition and Health Project (World Bank 1992) and Senegal's Community Nutrition Project (World Bank 2001b).

Question 5: Who gets how much?

The key variables here are coverage, intensity, quality, and targeting.

Coverage, intensity, and quality

Governments are often preoccupied with program coverage, both because they want to reach as many needy clients as possible and because of the political rewards of extending programs into new geographic areas. But when resources are scarce, there is a significant trade-off between a program's coverage and its intensity and quality. Intensity is measured by the amount of money spent per beneficiary, or the number of workers for a given client population. Mason and others (forthcoming) argue that to get a reasonable level of quality and impact, community nutrition programs need to spend in the range of $5–$10 a child per year, and have about one full-time worker (or a correspondingly larger number of part-time workers) for every 500 target families. Many programs have gone for high levels of coverage at the expense of intensity and quality. India's Integrated Child Development Services (ICDS) program, whose quality and impact is low, and which spends only about $2 a child per year on nutrition, is an example.

Targeting

There is therefore a trade-off, often unacknowledged, between getting a low-quality program to a large number of clients, and getting a higher quality program to a smaller number of clients. From an epidemiological and economic perspective, it is rational to target a higher-intensity, higher-quality program on limited geographic areas or high-risk population groups with high levels of malnutrition, rather than to seek universal, low-quality coverage. Targeting on the basis of highest need is not only equitable, but often the fastest way to get results because it is easier to reduce malnutrition from high to medium levels than from medium to low levels. For example, TINP, which was targeted on vulnerable children under age three, was able to reduce severe malnutrition from about 8 percent to about 4 percent in the first two years the program came into a new geographic area.

But while targeting high-intensity programs on the neediest may be epidemiologically and economically rational, benefiting only the most disadvantaged—who are seldom influential voters—may not be politically rational. The trade-off between tight targeting and political and community support can be resolved in various ways. In the case of TINP, a program in which food supplementation was tightly targeted on malnourished children under age three, only 25 percent of children received food

208 REPOSITIONING NUTRITION

supplementation at any given time; but because children whose growth
was faltering received supplementation, and because most children's growth
faltered at some time or other, 75 percent of children benefited from
supplementation at one time or another—thus ensuring wide community
support for the program (Heaver 2003a).

Question 6: How should things evolve over time?

If there aren't the funds to get adequate-intensity, adequate-quality programs to everyone, and if tight targeting on the neediest is politically difficult, another way to resolve this trade-off is to postpone more expensive,
higher-intensity interventions and concentrate in the short run on less costly
interventions that can reach more people. In practice, this usually means
concentrating on micronutrient programs (see Question 2), which can often
satisfy financial and political rationalities at the same time. Since micronutrient malnutrition is widespread and serious, these programs are an epidemiological priority too.

The problem is that PEM also has to be tackled in poor countries, where
it contributes to as many as half of child deaths, as well as to disease, low
school enrollment, and poor school performance. Because programs to promote child growth are those where many countries have invested least,
and since growth promotion programs are fairly expensive, deciding what
to do about PEM, and when, often presents the hardest of policy choices
for very poor countries. Four rules of thumb can be applied to help decide
how things should evolve over time.

Short-run plans should be pragmatic

Priorities for the next five years should be pragmatically determined, based
on a mix of criteria: what is epidemiologically important; what will get
political support; what is cost-effective and affordable; and what can be
implemented given existing management capacity, and taking into account
where past investment has gone and hence where there is a base for doing
more. Box 5.2 in the main volume of this report gives some examples of
what countries might do in the short run when commitment or financial
and managerial capacity are weak.

A long-term vision should be developed

This should set out the desired type and coverage of nutrition programs, and
the policies, institutions, commitment, capacity, and finance that need to
be put in place over a 10- to 15-year period to enable and support them.

Levels and trends in malnutrition and its causes (food insecurity, poor health, and inadequate caring practices) should be used to define what interventions are needed.

Foundations for the future should be laid

An implementable set of additional activities required to move the country along the path to its long-term vision should be built into the short-term plan. These might include policy analysis; building the data and evidence base; advocacy and alliance-building to strengthen commitment to the next generation of programs (see Heaver 2005b for details); and action research through small-scale projects to test service delivery strategies, and in particular to find out what intensity of resource use is required to reach an acceptable level of quality and impact.

Hard decisions about reorienting expenditures should not be ducked

The process of preparing PRSPs is supposed to facilitate prioritizing the actions that will do most to reduce poverty. But currently, though most PRSPs identify malnutrition as an important symptom of poverty, they either fail to include actions or budgets for improving nutrition; include funds only for micronutrient programs; or include as nutrition interventions actions such as school feeding that actually have little impact on nutrition (Shekar and Lee 2005).

Since malnutrition is both a major cause of income poverty and a key manifestation of poverty itself, if the PRSP process is to be meaningful, it should be used to reallocate resources from uses that have less impact on poverty to tackling malnutrition. This will mean working to ensure that:

• Items that do not do much to benefit nutrition are not included in the nutrition budget (for example, school feeding, which primarily benefits school enrollment, should be funded from the education and not the nutrition budget).
• Resources are reallocated from lower-impact indirect interventions to higher-impact PEM interventions targeted on high-risk groups if there is not enough government budget for both (for example, reallocations might be made from general food subsidies or from livelihood creation programs with no direct impact on food security and nutrition).
• Resources are reallocated to nutrition programs from other sectors with less direct impact on poverty (for example, by reducing power subsidies or selling state-owned manufacturing enterprises).

Annex 5.5
Methodology for constructing the country prioritization matrix

The construction of the matrix in figure 5.2 (see page 125) is based on the available prevalence data[2] for underweight (WAZ<2), stunting (HAZ<2), overweight (WHZ>2), iron deficiency anemia (IDA), and subclinical vitamin A deficiency (VAD) among children in World Bank client countries. Information on prevalence of wasting (WHZ<_2) and iodine deficiency disorders (IDD), measured by total goiter rate, is also included.

Out of 146 countries eligible for Bank financing, data are available from 126 countries for stunting and/or underweight, 82 countries have overweight data, and 80 countries have IDA and VAD data. Wasting and IDD data are available for 120 and 70 countries respectively. However, trend data are available for most countries only for underweight and stunting rates.

Cutoffs used to identify nutrition problems of public health significance

Category of public health significance	Stunting[a]	Under-weight	Wasting	Overweight[b]	IDA[c]	VAD[c]	IDD[c]
Severe	≥40	≥30	≥15	≥10	≥40	≥20	≥30
Moderate	30–39	20–29	10–14	5–9	20–39	10–20	20–29
Mild	20–29	10–19	5–9	3–4	5–19	2–9	5–19

[a]WHO (1995, 2000).
[b]By definition, only 2.3 percent of the children should have weight-for-height Z score >2. Countries with more than 1, 2, or 3 time(s) higher than this normal prevalence are, respectively, categorized as having mild, moderate, and severe levels of overweight.
[c]WHO (2000).

For the purposes of this prioritization of countries for action in nutrition, we used cut-offs corresponding to moderate malnutrition for underweight, wasting, IDA, VAD, and IDD. However, in view of the fact that stunting is an indicator of chronic undernutrition, and in view of the longer-term consequences of even mild stunting on economic productivity (see chapter 1), as well as the emerging nature of the noncommunicable disease (NCD) problem, we used lower cut-offs (corresponding to mild stunting and mild overweight) to identify countries where these agendas need to be pursued through development partner support. See figure 5.2 and accompanying text.

Annex 5.6
Nutritional status of children

Country	U5MR	Stunting	Underweight	Wasting	Overweight	VAD	IDA	IDD (TGR)	ARC* in stunting	ARC* in underweight
AFR										
Angola	260	45.2	30.5	6.3		55	72	33	-0.033	-0.057
Benin	151	30.7	22.9	7.5	1.3	70	82	4	0.041	-0.049
Botswana	110	23.1	12.5	5.0		30	37	17	-0.056	-0.080
Burkina Faso	207	36.8	34.3	13.2	1.6	46	83	29	0.017	0.008
Burundi	208	56.8	45.1	7.5	1.1	44	82	42		
Cameroon	166	29.3	22.2	5.9	2.9	36	58	12	0.017	0.055
Cape Verde	38	16.2	13.5	5.6						
Central African Rep.	180	28.4	23.2	6.4	0.8	68	74	11		-0.010
Chad	200	29.1	28.0	11.2		45	76	24	-0.107	-0.109
Comoros	79	42.3	26.0	11.5	3.8				0.031	0.031
Congo, DR	205	38.1	31.0	13.4		58	58		-0.028	-0.017
Congo, Rep.	108	27.5	23.9	5.5		32	55	36		
Côte d'Ivoire	191	25.1	21.2	7.8	1.5				0.006	-0.023
Equatorial Guinea	152									
Eritrea	80	37.6	39.6	12.6		30	75	10	-0.047	-0.007
Ethiopia	171	51.5	47.2	10.5		30	85	23	-0.028	0.003
Gabon	85	20.7	11.9	2.7		41	43	27	0.005	-0.008

Nutritional status of children (continued)

Country	U5MR	Stunting	Underweight	Wasting	Overweight	VAD	IDA	IDD (TGR)	ARC* in stunting	ARC* in underweight
Gambia, The	126	19.1	17.1	8.2		64	75	20	-0.114	-0.107
Ghana	97	25.9	24.9	9.5	1.9	60	65	18	0.000	-0.018
Guinea	165	41.0	33.0	9.1		40	73	23	0.041	0.034
Guinea-Bissau	211	30.4	25.0	10.3		31	83	17		
Kenya	122	33.0	22.1	6.1	3.5	70	60	10	-0.003	-0.008
Lesotho	132	45.4	17.8	5.4		54	51	19	0.045	0.003
Liberia	235	39.5	26.5	6.0		38	69	18		
Madagascar	135	48.6	33.1	7.4	1.0	42	73	6	-0.008	-0.023
Malawi	182	49.0	25.4	5.5	6.7	59	80	22	0.000	-0.013
Mali	222	38.2	33.2	10.6	1.3	47	77	42	-0.048	0.042
Mauritania	183	34.5	31.8	12.8		17	74	21	-0.050	-0.040
Mauritius	19	9.7	14.9	13.7	4.0					
Mozambique	205	35.9	26.1	7.9		26	80	17	-0.213	-0.017
Namibia	67	28.5	26.2	8.6	3.3	59	42	18		
Niger	264	39.7	40.1	13.6	1.1	41	57	20	0.002	0.000
Nigeria	201	33.5	30.7	15.6	3.3	25	69	8	-0.026	-0.019
Rwanda	203	42.6	24.3	6.8	2.1	39	69	13	-0.017	-0.024
São Tomé and Príncipe	118	28.9	12.9	3.6						
Senegal	138	25.4	22.7	8.4	2.6	61	71	23	-0.012	0.005
Seychelles	16	5.1	5.7	2.0	3.5					
Sierra Leone	284	33.8	27.2	9.9		47	86	16	-0.003	-0.005
Somalia	225	23.3	25.8	17.2						
South Africa	65	22.8	9.2	2.5	6.7	33	37	16	-0.108	
Sudan	94	34.3	40.7	13.1						0.026

Swaziland	149	30.2	10.3	1.3	2.5	38	47	12	0.002	0.003
Tanzania	165	43.8	29.4	5.4	2.5	37	65	16	-0.225	0.139
Togo	140	21.7	25.1	12.3	2.8	35	72	14	0.003	-0.019
Uganda	141	39.1	22.8	4.1	3.3	66	64	9	0.016	0.018
Zambia	182	46.8	28.1	5.0	4.2	66	63	25	0.043	-0.035
Zimbabwe	123	26.5	13.0	6.4		28	53	9		
EAP										
Cambodia	138	44.6	45.2	15.0	4.3	42	63	18	-0.045	-0.012
China	38	14.2	10.0	2.2	1.2	12	8	5	-0.111	-0.078
Fiji	21	2.7	7.9	8.2	4.0					
Indonesia	43	42.2	24.6		11.1	26	48	10	-0.024	-0.046
Kiribati	69	28.3	12.9	10.8						
Lao, PDR	100	40.7	40.0	15.4		42	54	14		-0.009
Malaysia	8		20.1							-0.047
Marshall Islands	66									
Micronesia, FS	24									
Mongolia	71	24.6	12.7	3.6	3.9	29	37	15	-0.010	0.003
Myanmar	108	41.6	28.2	8.2		35	48	17	0.007	-0.002
Palau	29									
Papua New Guinea	94	43.2	29.9	5.5	1.6	37	40	15	-0.017	-0.006
Philippines	37	32.1	31.8	6.5	0.8	23	29			
Samoa	25	3.8	4.2							
Solomon Islands	24	25.7	21.3	6.6	1.1					
Thailand	28	13.4	17.6	5.4	1.2	22	22	13	-0.089	-0.028
Timor-Leste	126	46.7	42.6							
Tonga	20	1.3		0.9					0.051	
Vanuatu	42	20.1	12.1	5.5					-0.045	
Vietnam	26	36.5	33.8	8.6	0.7	12	39	11		-0.029

Nutritional status of children (continued)

Country	U5MR	Stunting	Underweight	Wasting	Overweight	VAD	IDA	IDD (TGR)	ARC* in stunting	ARC* in underweight
ECA										
Albania	24	31.7	14.3	11.1	6.3				0.097	0.284
Armenia	35	12.9	2.6	1.9	3.7	12	24	12	0.017	-0.075
Azerbaijan	96	19.6	16.8	8.0		23	33	15	-0.031	0.127
Belarus	20									
Bosnia-Herzegovina	18	9.7	4.1	6.3						
Bulgaria	16									
Croatia	8	0.8	0.6	0.8	5.9				0.067	-0.077
Czech Republic	5	1.9	1.0	2.1	4.1					
Estonia	12									
Georgia	29	11.7	3.1	2.3		11	33	21		
Hungary	9	2.9	2.2	1.6	2.0					
Kazakhstan	99	9.7	4.2	1.8	4.3	19	49	21	-0.122	-0.170
Kyrgyz Republic	61	24.8	5.8	3.4		18	42	21		-0.160
Latvia	21									
Lithuania	9									
Macedonia, FYR	26	6.9	5.9	3.6	5.0					
Moldova	32									
Poland	9									
Romania	21	10.1	3.2	2.3	2.3				0.023	-0.060
Russian Federation	21	11.0	5.5						-0.074	0.054
Serbia and Montenegro	19	5.1	1.9						-0.072	0.043
Slovak Republic	9									
Tajikistan	116	30.9		4.9		18	45	28	0.000	

Country										
Turkey	41	16.0	8.3	1.9	2.9	18	23	23	-0.050	-0.047
Turkmenistan	86	22.3	12.0	5.7		18	36	11		
Ukraine	20	15.9	3.2	6.2						
Uzbekistan	65	31.3	18.8	11.6	14.4	40	33	24		
LAC										
Argentina	19	12.4	5.4	3.2	7.3				0.485	0.522
Belize	40		6.2							
Bolivia	71	26.8	7.6	1.3	6.5	23	59	4	0.000	-0.053
Brazil	37	10.5	5.7	2.3	4.9	15	45	4		
Chile	12	1.5	0.8	0.3	7.0		8		-0.121	-0.052
Colombia	23	13.5	6.7	0.8	2.6				-0.021	-0.045
Costa Rica	11	6.1	5.1	2.3	6.2					0.083
Dominica	15									
Dominican Republic	38	6.1	4.6	1.5	2.8	18	25	11	-0.110	-0.090
Ecuador	29	26.4	14.3	2.4	2.2					
El Salvador	39	18.9	10.3	1.4		17	28	11	-0.021	-0.008
Grenada										
Guatemala	49	46.4	24.2	2.5	4.0	21	34	16	-0.017	-0.024
Guyana	72	10.0	11.8	11.4	2.3					-0.046
Haiti	123	22.7	17.3	4.5	2.8	32	66	12	-0.040	-0.044
Honduras	42	29.2	16.6	1.1	1.4	15	34	12	-0.029	-0.008
Jamaica	20	4.4	3.8	3.8	6.0				-0.068	-0.061
Mexico	29	17.7	7.5	2.0	3.7				-0.217	-0.271
Nicaragua	41	20.2	9.6	2.0	2.8	9	47	4	-0.010	-0.013
Panama	25	18.2	8.1	1.0	3.7				0.122	0.057
Paraguay	30	13.9	3.7	0.3	3.9	13	52	13		
Peru	39	25.4	7.1	0.9	6.4	17	50	10	-0.028	-0.051
St. Kitts and Nevis	24									
St. Lucia	19	10.8	13.8	6.1	2.5					

Nutritional status of children (continued)

ARC* in Country	U5MR	Stunting	Underweight	Wasting	Overweight	VAD	IDA	IDD (TGR)	ARC* in stunting	ARC* in underweight
St. Vincent and the Grenadines	25	23.5	19.5	6.5						
Suriname	40	9.8	13.2	4.4						
Trinidad and Tobago	20	3.6	5.9		3.0					
Uruguay	15	9.5	4.4	1.4	6.2					
Venezuela	22	12.8	4.4	3.0	3.0	5	41	10	0.002	-0.032
MNA										
Algeria	49	18.0	6.0	2.7	9.2				-0.001	-0.063
Djibouti	143	25.7	18.2	12.9						
Egypt, Arab Rep. of	39	18.7	4.0	5.1	8.6	7	31	12	-0.045	-0.057
Iran, Islamic Rep. of	41	15.4	10.9	4.9	3.3	23	32	9	-0.068	-0.122
Iraq	125	22.1	15.9	5.9					0.002	0.032
Jordan	33	7.8	5.1	1.9	5.7				-0.101	-0.033
Lebanon	32	12.2	3.0	2.9		20	21	11	-0.009	-0.011
Morocco	43	23.1	9.5	2.2	6.8	29	45		-0.044	-0.089
Syrian Arab Republic	28	18.8	6.9	3.8		8	40	8		
Tunisia	26	12.3	4.0	2.2	3.5				-0.101	-0.148
Yemen, Rep. of	114	51.7	46.1	12.9	4.3	40	59	16	0.024	0.061
SAR										
Afghanistan	257	47.6	49.3	16.1	4.0	53	65	48		
Bangladesh	73	44.7	47.7	10.3	1.1	28	55	18	-0.030	-0.023
Bhutan	94	40.0	18.7	2.6	2.0	32	81			
India	90	44.9	46.7	15.7	1.6	57	75	26	-0.024	-0.024
Maldives	77	36.0	45.0	20.0	1.2				0.060	0.031

Nepal	83	50.5	48.3	9.6	0.5	33	65	24	-0.016	0.001
Pakistan	101	36.3	38.2	14.2	3.1	35	56	38	-0.104	-0.005
Sri Lanka	19	20.4	32.9	13.3	0.1				-0.077	-0.015

ARC=Annual rate of change.
See also Figure 2.12 and Maps 1.1–1.4

Notes

1. Epidemiology, cost-effectiveness, commitment, capacity, affordability, where past investment has gone, who should benefit, coverage, intensity, timing.

2. Stunting, underweight, wasting, IDD data from SCN (2004). VAD and IDA data from UNICEF and MI (2004b). Overweight data from De Onis and Blossner (2000).

References

ACC/SCN (Administrative Committee on Coordination/Subcommittee on Nutrition of the United Nations). 1997. "Effective Programmes in Africa for Improving Nutrition, Including Household Food Security." Symposium Report. *SCN News* 15. Geneva.

ACC/SCN. 2000. *Low birthweight: Report of a Meeting in Dhaka, Bangladesh on 14–17 June 1999*, ed. J. Pojda and L. Kelley, Nutrition Policy Paper #18. Geneva: ACC/SCN in collaboration with ICDDR,B.

Acharya, Karabi, Tina Sanghvi, Serigne Diene, Vandana Stapleton, Eleonore Seumo, Sridhar Srikantiah, and others. 2004. *Using 'Essential Nutrition Actions' (ENA) to Accelerate Coverage with Nutrition Interventions in High Mortality Settings*. Published for the U.S. Agency for International Development by the Basic Support for Institutionalizing Child Survival (BASICS II) Project, Arlington, VA.

Adams, R.H. 1998. "The Political Economy of the Food Subsidy System in Bangladesh." *Journal of Development Studies* 35(1): 66–88.

AED (Academy for Educational Development). 2003. PROFILES: Summary of assessment findings and future directions. Available at http://www.aedprofiles.org/media/publications/PROFILES%20EVALUATION%20BRIEF.pdf.

Aguayo, V.M., S.K. Baker, X. Crespin, H. Hamani, and A. Mamadoultaibou. 2005. "Maintaining High Vitamin A Supplementation Coverage in Children: Lessons from Niger." New York: Helen Keller International Africa, Nutrition in Development Series, Issue 5.

Alderman, Harold. 2002. "Subsidies as a Social Safety Net: Effectiveness and Challenges." Washington, DC: World Bank, Social Protection Discussion Paper 0224.

Alderman, Harold, and Jere R. Behrman. 2004. "Estimated Economic Benefits of Reducing Low Birth Weight in Low-Income Countries." Washington, DC: World Bank HNP Discussion Paper.

Alderman, Harold, and Kathy Lindert. 1998. "The Potential and Limitations of Self-Targeted Food Subsidies." Oxford: Oxford University Press. *World Bank Research Observer* 13(2): 213–29.

Alderman, Harold, J.G.M. (Hans) Hoogeveen, and Mariacristina Rossi. 2005. "Reducing Child Malnutrition in Tanzania: Combined Effects of Income Growth and Program Interventions." Washington, DC: World Bank Policy Research Working Paper 3567.

Allen, Lindsay H., and Stuart R. Gillespie. 2001. *What Works? A Review of the Efficacy and Effectiveness of Nutrition Interventions*. Geneva: United Nations Administrative Committee on Coordination Subcommittee on Nutrition, Asian Development Bank, and International Food Policy Research Institute.

Anderson, M.A. 1981. "Health and Nutrition Impact of Potable Water in Rural Bolivia." *Journal of Tropical Pediatrics* 27: 39–46.

Attanasio, Orazio, Erich Battistin, Elma Fitzsimons, Alice Mesnard, and Marcos Vera-Hernández. 2005. "How Effective Are Conditional Cash Transfers? Evidence from Colombia." London: The Institute for Fiscal Studies, Briefing Note No. 54.

Barker, David J.P. 2002. "Fetal Programming of Coronary Heart Disease." *Trends in Endocrinology and Metabolism* 13(9): 364–8.

———. 2004. "The Developmental Origins of Well-Being." *Philosophical Transactions of the Royal Society of London*. Series B, Biological Sciences. 3591449: 1359–66.

Barker, David J.P., Johan G. Eriksson, T. Forsén, and Clive Osmond. 2002. "Fetal Origins of Adult Disease: Strength of Effects and Biological Basis." *International Journal of Epidemiology* 31(6): 1235–39.

Barker, David J.P., T.W. Meade, C.H. Fall, A. Lee, C.K. Phipps, and Y. Stirling. 1992. "Relation of Fetal and Infant Growth to Plasma Fibrinogen and Factor VII Concentrations in Adult Life." *British Medical Journal* 304(6820): 148–52.

Barros, F.C., and J.S. Robinson. 2000. "Addressing low birthweight through interventions in pregnancy." Technical consultation on low birthweight. New York: Jointly organized by the U.S. Department of Agriculture, the Human Development Network of the World Bank, and UNICEF.

Beaton, George H., R. Martorell, K.J. Aronson, B. Edmonston, G. McCabe, A.C. Ross, and B. Harvey. 1993. "Effectiveness of Vitamin A Supplementation in the Control of Young Child Morbidity and Mortality in Developing Countries." Geneva: The United Nations, Administrative Committee on Coordination/Subcommittee on Nutrition State-of-the-Art Series, Nutrition Policy Discussion Paper 13.

Behrman, Jere R., and John Hoddinott. 2001. "An Evaluation of the Impact of PROGRESA on Preschool Child Height." Washington, DC: International Food Policy Research Institute FCND Discussion Paper 104.

Behrman, Jere R., and Mark R. Rosenzweig. 2001. "The Returns to Increasing Body Weight." Philadelphia: Penn Institute for Economic Research, Working Paper 01-052. Available at http://ssrn.com/abstract=297919.

Behrman, Jere R., Harold Alderman, and John Hoddinott. 2004. "Nutrition and Hunger." In *Global Crises, Global Solutions*, ed. Bjorn Lomborg. Cambridge, UK: Cambridge University Press.

Berg, Alan. 1987. *Malnutrition: What Can Be Done? Lessons from World Bank Experience*. Baltimore and London: Johns Hopkins University Press for the World Bank.

————. 1992. "Sliding toward Nutrition Malpractice: Time to Reconsider and Redeploy." *American Journal of Clinical Nutrition* 57: 3–7.

Bhagwati, Jagdish, Robert Fogel, Bruno Frey, Justin Yifu Lin, Douglass North, Thomas Schelling, and others. 2004. "Ranking the Opportunities." In *Global Crises, Global Solutions*, ed. Bjorn Lomborg. Cambridge, UK: Cambridge University Press.

Bhargava, S.K., H.P.S. Sachdev, C.H. Fall, Clive Osmond, R. Lakshmy, David J.P. Barker, and others. 2004. "Relation of serial changes in childhood body mass index to impaired glucose tolerance in young adulthood." *New England Journal of Medicine* 350: 865–75.

Bryce, J., C. Boschi-Pinto, K. Shibuya, Robert E. Black, and the WHO Child Health Epidemiology Reference Group. 2005. "New WHO Estimates of the Causes of Child Deaths." *Lancet* 365: 1147–52.

Burger, S.E. and Steven A. Esrey. 1995. "Water and Sanitation: Health and Nutrition Benefits to Children." In *Child Growth and Nutrition in Developing Countries: Priorities for Action*, ed. Per Pinstrup-Andersen, David Pelletier, and Harold Alderman, Ithaca, NY: Cornell University Press.

Caballero, B. 2005. "A nutrition paradox—underweight and obesity in developing countries." *N Engl J Med* 352(15): 1514–1516.

Cairncross, Sandy, and Vivian Valdimanis. 2004. "Water Supply, Sanitation, and Hygiene Promotion." Fogarty International Center, Disease Control Priorities Project Working Paper 28. Bethesda, MD: National Institutes of Health. Available at www.fic.nih.gov/dcpp.

Caldes, Natalia, David Coady, and John A. Maluccio. 2004. "The Cost of Poverty Alleviation Transfer Programs: A Comparative Analysis of Three Programs in Latin America." Washington, DC: International Food Policy Research Institute FCND Discussion Paper 174.

Carroll, Amy, Lisa Craypo, and Sarah E. Samuels. 2000. "Evaluating Nutrition and Physical Activity Social Marketing Campaigns: A Review of the Literature for Use in Community Campaigns." A Report to the Center for Advanced Studies of Nutrition and Social Marketing, University of California, Davis.

Caulfield, Laura E., Stephanie A. Richard, and Robert E. Black. 2004. "Undernutrition As an Underlying Cause of Malaria Morbidity and Mortality in Children Less Than Five Years Old." *American Journal of Tropical Medicine and Hygiene* 71(Supplement 2): 55–63.

Caulfield, Laura E., Mercedes de Onis, Monika Blössner, and Robert E. Black. 2004a. "Undernutrition as an Underlying Cause of Child Deaths Associated with Diarrhea, Pneumonia, Malaria, and Measles." *American Journal of Clinical Nutrition* 80: 193–98.

Caulfield, Laura E., Stephanie A. Richard, Juan A. Rivera, Philip Musgrove, and Robert E. Black. 2004b. "Stunting, Wasting, and Micronutrient Deficiency Disorders." Version of 23 December 2004, prepared for Disease Control Priorities in Developing Countries, second edition (DCP2).

Chen, Jun-shi, X. Zhao, X. Zhang, S. Yin, J. Pioa, J. Huo, and others. 2005. "Studies on the Effectiveness of NaFeEDTA-fortified Soy Sauce for Controlling Iron Deficiency: A Population-Based Intervention Trial." *Food and Nutrition Bulletin* 26(2): 177–86.

Chen and Ravallion. 2004. "How Have the World's Poor Fared since the Early 1980s?" Washington, DC: World Bank Research Observer 19(2).

Chhabra, Ritu, and Claudia Rokx. 2004. "The Nutrition MDG Indicator: Interpreting Progress." Washington, DC: World Bank HNP Discussion Paper.

Christiaensen, Luc, and Harold Alderman. 2004. "Child Malnutrition in Ethiopia: Can Maternal Knowledge Augment the Role of Income?" *Economic Development and Cultural Change* 52(2): 287–312.

Christian, Parul, Subarna K. Khatry, Joanne Katz, Elizabeth K. Pradhan, Steven C. LeClerq, Sharada Ram Shrestha, and others. 2003. "Effects of Alternative Maternal Micronutrient Supplements on Low Birth Weight in Rural Nepal: Double Blind Randomized Community Trial." *British Medical Journal* 326:571.

Coady, David. 2003. "Alleviating Structural Poverty in Developing Countries: The Approach of PROGRESA in Mexico." Washington, DC: International Food Policy Research Institute, IFPRI Perspectives, Vol. 23.

Coleman, Karen J., and Eugenia C. Gonzalez. 2001."Promoting stair use in a U.S.-Mexico border community." *American Journal of Public Health* 91: 2007–9.

Coleman, Karen J., Claire Lola Tiller, Jesus Sanchez, Edward M. Heath, Oumar Sy, George Milliken, and David A. Dzewaltowski. 2005. "Prevention of the epidemic increase in child risk of overweight in low-income schools." *Archives of Pediatric & Adolescent Medicine* 159: 217–24.

Coutsoudis Anna, Kubendran Pillay, Elizabeth Spooner, Louise Kuhn, and Hoosen M. Coovadia. 1999. "Influence of Infant-Feeding Patterns on Early Mother-to-Child Transmission of HIV-1 in Durban, South Africa: A Prospective Cohort Study." *Lancet* 354: 471–76.

Coutsoudis, Anna, François Dabis, Wafaie Fawzi, Philippe Gaillard, Geert Haverkamp, D.R. Harris, and others and The Breastfeeding and HIV International Transmission Study Group (BHITS). 2004. "Late Postnatal

Transmission of HIV-1 in Breast-Fed Children: An Individual Patient Data Meta-Analysis." *Journal of Infectious Diseases* 189 (12): 2154–66.

Darnton-Hill, I., P. Webb, P.W.J. Harvey, and others. 2005. "Micronutrient deficiencies and gender: social and economic costs." *Am J Clin Nutr* 81(S): 1198S–1205S.

De Onis, Mercedes, and Monika Blössner. 2000. "Prevalence and Trends of Overweight among Preschool Children in Developing Countries." *American Journal of Clinical Nutrition* 72: 1032–39.

De Onis, Mercedes, Monika Blössner, Elaine Borghi, Richard Morris, and Edward Frongillo. 2004a. "Methodology for estimating regional and global trends of child malnutrition." *International Journal of Epidemiology* 33: 1260–70.

De Onis, Mercedes, Monika Blössner, Elaine Borghi, Edward Frongillo, and Richard Morris. 2004b. "Estimates of Global Prevalence of Childhood Underweight in 1990 and 2015." *Journal of the American Medical Association* 291(21): 2600–06.

Deitchler, Megan, Ellen Mathys, John Mason, Pattanee Winichagoon, and Ma Antonia Tuazon. 2004. "Lessons from Successful Micronutrient Programs. Part II: Program Implementation." *Food and Nutrition Bulletin* 25(1): 30–95.

Delisle, Hélène, V. Chandra-Mouli, and Bruno de Benoist. 2000 (posted). "Should Adolescents Be Specifically Targeted for Nutrition in Developing Countries: To Address Which Problems, and How?" World Health Organization/International Nutrition Foundation for Developing Countries. Available at http://www.who.int/child-adolescent-health/New_Publications/NUTRITION/Adolescent_nutrition_paper.pdf.

Diagana, Bocar, Francis Akindes, Kimseyinga Savadogo, Thomas Reardon, and John Staatz. 1999. "Effects of the CFA Franc Devaluation on Urban Food Consumption in West Africa: Overview and Cross-Country Comparisons." *Food Policy* 24: 465–78.

Dickin, K., M. Griffiths, and E. Piwoz. 1997. "Designing by Dialogue: A Program Planners' Guide to Consultative Research for Improving Young Child Feeding." Washington, DC: Health and Human Resources Analysis Project, The Manoff Group, Support for Analysis and Research in Africa. Available at http://sara.aed.org/publications/child_survival/nutrition/dbyd_feeding/D%20by%20D_Feed%20(full).pdf.

Doak, Colleen M. 2002. "Large-Scale Interventions and Programmes Addressing Nutrition-Related Chronic Diseases and Obesity: Examples from 14 Countries." *Public Health Nutrition* 5(1A): 275–77.

Doak, Colleen M., L.S. Adair, M. Bentley, C. Monteiro, and Barry M. Popkin. 2005. "The Dual Burden Household and the Nutrition Transition Paradox." *International Journal of Obesity* 29: 129–36.

Dolan, Carmel, and F. James Levinson. 2000. "Will We Ever Get Back? The Derailing of Tanzanian Nutrition in the 1990s." Washington, DC and New York: Draft paper submitted for the World Bank-UNICEF Nutrition Assessment. Processed.

Dowda, Marsha, James F. Sallis, Thomas L. McKenzie, Paul Rosengard, and Harold W. Kohl III. 2005. "Evaluating the Sustainability of SPARK Physical Education: A Case Study of Translating Research into Practice." *Research Quarterly for Exercise and Sport* 76: 11–19.

Elmendorf, Edgard A., Cecilia Cabanero-Verzosa, Michèle Lioy, and Kathryn LaRusso. 2005. "Behavior Change Communication for Better Health Outcomes in Africa: Experience and Lessons learned from World Bank Financed Health, Nutrition, and Population Projects." Washington DC: Africa Region Human Development Working Paper Series No. 52.

Eriksson, Johan G., T. Forsén, J. Tuomilehto, Clive Osmond, and David J.P. Barker. 2001. "Early Growth and Coronary Heart Disease in Later Life: Longitudinal Study." *British Medical Journal* 322: 949–53.

Esanu, Cristina, and Kathy Lindert. 1996. "An Analysis of Consumer Food Price and Subsidy Policies in Romania." Washington, DC: World Bank ASAL Unit, Romania.

Ezzati, Majid, Alan Lopez, Anthony Rodgers, Stephen Vander Hoorn, Christopher Murray, and the Comparative Risk Assessment Collaborating Group. 2002. "Selected Major Risk Factors and Global and Regional Burden of Disease." *Lancet* 360(9343): 1–14.

FANTA (Food and Nutrition Technical Assistance Project). 2004. "HIV/AIDS: A Guide for Nutritional Care and Support." 2nd Edition. Food and Nutrition Technical Assistance Project. Washington, DC: Academy for Educational Development.

FAO Statistical Database Data. 2005. Last updated on Aug 22, 2004. http://faostat.fao.org/faostat/collections?subset=nutrition.

Fawzi, Waifaie, Gernard Msamanga, Donna Spiegelman, and David J. Hunter. 2005. "Studies of Vitamins and Minerals and HIV Transmission and Disease Progression." *Journal of Nutrition* 135: 938–44.

Fawzi, Waifaie, Gernard Msamanga, Donna Spiegelman, R. Wei, S. Kapiga, E. Villamor, and others. 2004. "A Randomized Trial of Multivitamin Supplements and HIV Disease Progression and Mortality." *New England Journal of Medicine* 351: 23–32.

Fernald, Lia. 2005. "Obesity and Chronic Disease in the Developing World." Washington, DC: World Bank Background Paper.

Fewtrell, L., and J. Colford. 2004. "Water, Sanitation and Hygiene Interventions, and Diarrhoea: A Systematic Review and Meta-Analysis." Washington DC: World Bank Health, Nutrition, and Population Discussion Paper.

Fiedler, John L. 2000. "The Nepal National Vitamin A Program: Prototype to Emulate or Donor Enclave?" Health Policy and Planning 15(2): 145–56.

————. 2003. "A Cost Analysis of the Honduras Community-Based, Integrated Child Care Program (Atención Integral a la Niñez–Comunitaria, AIN-C). Washington, DC: World Bank HNP Discussion Paper.

Fiedler, John L., D.R. Dado, H. Maglalang, N. Juban, M. Capistrano, and M. V. Magpantay. 2000. "Cost Analysis As a Vitamin A Program Design and Evaluation Tool: A Case Study of the Philippines." Social Science and Medicine 51: 223–42.

Galloway, Rae. 2003. "Anemia Prevention and Control: What Works." A joint product of the Food and Agriculture Organization, the Micronutrient Initiative, the Pan American Health Organization, UNICEF, the U.S. Agency for International Development, the World Bank, and the World Health Organization.

Gastein Opinion Group. 2002. "Health at the Heart of CAP: Health and Common Agricultural Policy Reform Opinion and Proposals of an Expert Working Group." Gastein, Austria: European Health Policy Forum.

Gertler, Paul. 2000. "Final Report: The Impact of PROGRESA on Health." Washington, DC: International Food Policy Research Institute, Food Consumption and Nutrition Division. Available at ww.ifpri.org/themes/progresa/pdf/Gertler_health.pdf.

Gillespie, Stuart R. 2001. "Strengthening Capacity to Improve Nutrition." Washington, DC: International Food Policy Research Institute, FCND Discussion Paper 106.

————. 2004. "Scaling Up Community Driven Development: A Synthesis of Experience." Washington, DC: World Bank Social Development Paper 69.

Gillespie, Stuart R. 2002 "Nutrition in Transition." Washington DC: International Food Policy Research Institute, New and Noteworthy in Nutrition Issue No. 36:7.

Gillespie, Stuart R., and Lawrence Haddad. 2003. "The Relationship between Nutrition and the Millennium Development Goals: A Strategic Review of the Scope for DFID's Influencing Role." London: U.K. Department for International Development.

Gillespie, Stuart R., and Suneetha Kadiyala. 2005. "HIV/AIDS and Food and Nutrition Security: From Evidence to Action." Washington, DC: International Food Policy Research Institute, Food Policy Review No. 7.

Gillespie, Stuart R., John Mason, and Reynaldo Martorell. 1996. "How Nutrition Improves." Geneva: The United Nations, Administrative

Committee on Coordination/Subcommittee on Nutrition State-of-the-Art Series, Nutrition Policy Discussion Paper 15.

Gillespie, Stuart R., Milla McLachlan, and Roger Shrimpton, eds. 2003. *Combating Malnutrition: Time to Act.* Health, Nutrition, and Human Development Series. Washington, DC: World Bank.

Gragnolati, Michele, M. Shekar, M. Dasgupta, C. Bredenkamp, and Y.K. Lee. Forthcoming. *The Challenge of Persistent Child Undernutrition in India and the Role of the ICDS Program.* Washington, DC: World Bank.

Grantham-McGregor, Sally, Lia Fernald, and K. Sethurahman. 1999. "Effects of Health and Nutrition on Cognitive and Behavioural Development in Children in the First Three Years of Life." Food and Nutrition Bulletin 20(1): 53–99.

Griffiths, M., and J.S. McGuire. "A New Dimension for Health Reform: The Integrated Community Child Health Program in Honduras." 2005. In *Health System Innovations in Central America: Lessons and Impact of New Approaches,* ed. Gerard La Forgia. Washington, DC: World Bank Working Paper 57.

Gwatkin, D.R., S. Rutstein, K. Johnson, E.A. Suliman, and A. Wagstaff. 2003. *Initial Country-Level Information about Socio-Economic Differences in Health, Nutrition, and Population.* 2nd edition. Washington, DC: World Bank.

Habicht, Jean-Pierre, C.G. Victora, and J.P. Vaughan. 1999. "Evaluation Designs for Adequacy, Plausibility, and Probability of Public Health Programme Performance and Impact." *International Journal of Epidemiology* 28: 10–18.

Haddad, Lawrence. 2003. "Redirecting the Nutrition Transition: What Can Food Policy Do?" In "Food Policy Options: Preventing and Controlling Nutrition-Related Noncommunicable Diseases." World Health Organization and World Bank HNP Discussion Paper, Washington, DC: World Bank.

Haddad, Lawrence, and Lisa C. Smith. 1999. "Explaining Child Malnutrition in Developing Countries: A Cross-Country Analysis." Washington, DC: International Food Policy and Research Institute Discussion Paper 60.

Haddad, Lawrence, Harold Alderman, Simon Appleton, Lina Song, and Yisehac Yohannes. 2002. "Reducing Child Undernutrition: How Far Does Income Growth Take Us?" Washington, DC: International Food Policy Research Institute FCND Discussion Paper 137.

Haddad, Lawrence, Saroj Bhattarai, Maarten Immink, Shubh Kuman, and Alison Slack. 1995. "More Than Food Is Needed to Achieve Good Nutrition by 2020." Washington, DC: International Food Policy and Research Institute 2020 Vision Brief 25.

Haddad, Lawrence, Christine Pena, Chiruzu Nishida, Agnes Quisumbing, and Alison Slack. 1996. "Food Security and Nutrition Implications of

Intrahousehold Bias: A Review of Literature." Washington, DC: International Food Policy Research Institute FCND Discussion Paper 19.

Handa, Sudhanshu, and Mari-Carmen Huerta. 2004. "Using Clinic-Based Data to Estimate the Impact of a Nutrition Intervention." www.unc.edu/~shanda/research/ Handa_Huerta_Program_Bias_V1.pdf.

Hawkes, Corinna, Cara Eckhardt, Marie T. Ruel, and Nicholas Minot. 2005. "Diet Quality, Poverty, and Food Policy: A New Research Agenda for Obesity Prevention in Developing Countries." SCN News 29: 20–22, special issue: *Overweight and obesity: a new nutrition emergency?*

Heaver, Richard. 2002. "Improving Nutrition: Issues in Management and Capacity Development." Washington, DC: World Bank Health, Nutrition, and Population Discussion Paper.

————. 2003a. "India's Tamil Nadu Nutrition Program: Lessons and Issues in Management and Capacity Development." Washington, DC: World Bank Health, Nutrition, and Population Discussion Paper.

————. 2003b. "Nutrition and Community-Driven Development: Opportunities and Risks." Washington, DC: World Bank Social Development Notes 89.

————. 2005a. "Good Work—But Not Enough of It: A Review of the World Bank's Experience in Nutrition." Washington, DC: World Bank.

————. 2005b. "Strengthening Country Commitment to Human Development: Lessons from Nutrition." Washington, DC: World Bank Directions in Development Series.

Heaver, Richard, and Yongyout Kachondam. 2002. "Thailand's National Nutrition Program: Lessons in Management and Capacity Development." Washington, DC: World Bank HNP Discussion Paper.

Hendricks, Michael, Romy Saitowitz, and John Fiedler. 1998. "An Economic Analysis of Vitamin A Interventions in South Africa." Photocopy. Child Health Unit, University of Cape Town.

Hill, Zelee, Betty Kirkwood, and Karen Edmond. 2004. "Family and Community Practices That Promote Child Survival, Growth, and Development: A Review of the Evidence." Geneva: World Health Organization.

Ho, T.J. 1985. "Economic Issues in Assessing Nutrition Projects: Costs, Affordability, and Cost Effectiveness." Washington, DC: World Bank PHN Technical Note 85-14.

Hoddinott, John, and Emmanual Skoufias. 2003. "The Impact of PRO-GRESA on Food Consumption." Washington DC: International Food Policy Research Institute FCND Discussion Paper 150.

Honorati, M., J. Armstrong Schellenberg, H. Mshinda, M. Shekar, J.K.L. Mugyabuso, G.D. Ndossi, and D. de Savigny. Forthcoming. "Vitamin

A Supplementation in Tanzania: The Impact of a Change in Programmatic Delivery Strategy on Coverage."

Horton, Susan. 1993. "Cost Analysis of Feeding and Food Subsidy Programmes." *Food Policy* 18(3)192–99.

―――. 1999. "The Economics of Nutritional Interventions." In *Nutrition and Health in Developing Countries*, ed. Richard D. Semba and Martin W. Bloem. Totowa, NJ: Humana Press, Inc.

Horton, Susan, and J. Ross. 2003. "The Economics of Iron Deficiency." *Food Policy* 28(1): 51–75.

Horton, Susan, Tina Sanghvi, Margaret Phillips, John Fiedler, Rafael Perez-Escamilla, Chessa Lutter, Ada Rivera, and A.M. Segall-Correa. 1996. "Breastfeeding Promotion and Priority Setting in Health." *Health Policy Planning* 11(2):156–68.

Hunt, J.M. 2005. "The Potential Impact of Reducing Global Malnutrition on Poverty Reduction and Economic Development." Asia Pac J Clin Nutr 14(S): 10–38.

Hunt, Joseph Michael M., and M.G. Quibria. 1999. Investing in Child Nutrition in Asia. Manila: Asian Development Bank and UNICEF, ADB Nutrition and Development Series 1.

Iannotti, Lora, and Stuart Gillespie. 2002. *Successful Community Nutrition Programming: Lessons from Kenya, Tanzania, and Uganda.* New York: UNICEF.

Iliadou, Anastasia, Sven Cnattingius, and P. Lichtenstein. 2004. "Low Birthweight and Type 2 Diabetes: A Study on 11,162 Swedish Twins." *International Journal of Epidemiology* 33(5): 948–53.

Iliff, Peter J., Ellen G. Piwoz, Naume V. Tavengwa, Clare D. Zunguza, Edmore T. Marinda, Kusum J. Nathoo, and others. 2005. "Early Exclusive Breastfeeding Reduces the Risk of Postnatal HIV-1 Transmission and Increases HIV-Free Survival." *AIDS* 19(7): 699–708.

IASO (International Association for the Study of Obesity). 2004. *Global obesity epidemic putting brakes on economic development.* Available at http://www.iotf.org/media/releaseoct28.htm.

IFPRI (International Food Policy Research Institute). 2003. "Going after the Agriculture-Nutrition Advantage." *IFPRI Forum* September 2003. Only page number available: Pg. 7

International Obesity Task Force. 2003. International Obesity Task Force Press Statement. [http://www.iotf.org/media/iotfaug25.htm]. Accessed on 05/06/05.

Jennings, J., Stuart Gillespie, J. Mason, Mashed Lotfi, and T. Scialfa. 1991. *Managing Successful Nutrition Programs.* Geneva: The United Nations, Administrative Committee on Coordination, Subcommittee on Nutrition, Nutrition Policy Discussion Paper 8.

Johnston, Timothy, and Susan Stout. 1999. *Investing in Health: Development Effectiveness in the Health, Nutrition, and Population Sector.* Washington, DC: World Bank Operations Evaluation Department Report.

Jolly, R. 1996. Kenya: Our Planet: Poverty, Health, and the Environment. *Nutrition.* UNEP. Can be accessed at http://www.ourplanet.com/imgversn/122/jolly.html

Jones, Gareth, Richard W. Steketee, Robert E. Black, Zulfiqar A. Bhutta, Saul S. Morris, and the Bellagio Child Survival Study Group. 2003. "How Many Child Deaths Can We Prevent This Year?" *Lancet* 362: 65–71.

Jonsson, Urban. 1997. "Success Factors in Community-Based Nutrition-Oriented Programmes and Projects." In *Malnutrition in South Asia: A Regional Profile,* ed. Stuart Gillespie. Katmandu, Nepal: UNICEF Regional Office for South Asia.

Kahn, Emily B., Leigh T. Ramsey, Ross C. Brownson, Gregory W. Heath, Elizabeth H. Howze, Kenneth E. Powell, and others. 2002. "The Effectiveness of Interventions to Increase Physical Activity: A Systematic Review." *American Journal of Preventive Medicine* 22(4S): 73–107.

Kimm, Sue. 2004. "Fetal Origins of Adult Disease: The Barker Hypothesis Revisited—2004." *Current Opinion in Endocrinology & Diabetes* 11(4): 192–96.

Lee, Min-June, B.M. Popkin, and S. Kim. 2002. "The Unique Aspects of the Nutrition Transition in South Korea: The Retention of Healthful Elements in Their Traditional Diet." *Public Health Nutrition* 5(1a): 197–203.

Leith, Jennifer, Catherine Porter, SMERU Institute, and Peter Warr. 2003. Indonesia Rice Tariff Reform. On World Bank's PSIA website. Can be accessed at: http://web.worldbank.org/WBSITE/EXTERNAL/TOPICS/EXTPOVERTY/EXTPSIA/0,,contentMDK:20490211~menuPK:1108036~pagePK:148956~piPK:216618~theSitePK:490130,00.html

Levinson, James. 2002. "Searching for a Home: The Institutionalization Issue in International Nutrition." Washington, DC and New York: World Bank–UNICEF Nutrition Assessment Background Paper. Processed.

Maluccio, John A., and Rafael Flores. 2004. "Impact Evaluation of a Conditional Cash Transfer Program: The Nicaraguan *Red de Protección Social.*" Washington, DC: International Food Policy Research Institute FCND Discussion Paper 184.

Mannar, Venkatest, and Erick Boy Gallego. 2002. "Iron Fortification: Country Level Experiences and Lessons Learned." *Journal of Nutrition* 132: 856S–858S.

Mannar, Venkatest, and R. Shankar. 2004. "Micronutrient Fortification of Foods—Rationale, Application, and Impact." *Indian Journal of Pediatrics* 71: 997–1002.

Manoff International, Inc. 1984. *Nutrition Communication and Behavior Change Component: Indonesian Nutrition Development Program. Volume IV: Household Evaluation.* New York: Manoff International, Inc.

Marsh, David R., and David G. Schroeder, eds. 2002. "The Positive Deviance Approach to Improve Health Outcomes: Experience and Evidence from the Field." *Food and Nutrition Bulletin* 23(4, Supplement): 3–6.

Martorell, Reynaldo, K.L. Khan, and Dirk Schroeder. 1994. "Reversibility of Stunting: Epidemiological Findings in Children from Developing Countries." *European Journal of Clinical Nutrition* 48(Supplement): S45–S57.

Mason, John B., Philip Musgrove, and Jean-Pierre Habicht. 2003. "At Least One-Third of Poor Countries' Disease Burden Is Due to Malnutrition." Bethesda, MD: National Institutes of Health, Fogarty International Center, Disease Control Priorities Project Working Paper 1.

Mason, John B., Joseph Hunt, David Parker, and Urban Jonsson. 2001. "Improving Child Nutrition in Asia." Manila: Asian Development Bank. ADB Nutrition and Development Series 3.

Mason, John B., R. Galloway, J. Martines, Philip Musgrove, and D. Sanders. Forthcoming. "Community Health and Nutrition Programs." In *Disease Control Priorities in Developing Countries*, ed. Dean Jamison, George Alleyne, Joel Breman, Mariam Claeson, David Evans, Prabhat Jha, and others. 2nd edition. Oxford and New York: Oxford University Press for the World Bank.

Matsudo, S., D. Andrade, T. Araujo, E. Andrade, L.C. de Oliveira, G. Braggion, and S. Matsudo. 2002. "Promotion of Physical Activity in a Developing Country: The Agita Sao Paulo Experience. *Public Health Nutrition* 5(1A): 253–61.

Matta, Nadim, Ronald Ashkenas, and Jean-François Rischard. 2000. *Building Client Capacity through Results.* Washington, DC: World Bank Internal Report.

Matte, Thomas D, Michaeline Bresnahan, Melissas Begg, and Ezra Susser. 2001. "Influence of Variation in Birth Weight within Normal Range and within Sibships on IQ at Age 7 Years: Cohort Study." *British Medical Journal* 323(7308): 310–14.

Miura, Katsuyuki, H. Nakagawa, M. Tabata, Y. Morikawa, M. Nishijo, and S. Kagamimori. 2001. "Birth Weight, Childhood Growth, and Cardiovascular Disease Risk Factors in Japanese Aged 20 Years." *American Journal of Epidemiology* 153(8): 783–89.

Monteiro, Carlos A., Wolney L. Conde, B. Lu, and Barry M. Popkin. 2004. "Obesity and Inequities in Health in the Developing World." *International Journal of Obesity* 28: 1181–86.

Mora, José O., and Josefina Bonilla. 2002. "Successful Vitamin A Supplementation in Nicaragua." Basel, Switzerland: MOST (the United

States Agency for International Development Micronutrient Program) Newsletter 3.

Morris, Saul, Pedro Olinto, Rafael Flores, Eduardo A.F. Nilson, and Ana C. Figueiro. 2004. "Conditional Cash Transfers Are Associated with a Small Reduction in the Rate of Weight Gain of Preschool Children in Northeast Brazil." *Journal of Nutrition* 134 (9): 2336–42.

Neiman, Andrea B., and Enrique R. Jacoby. 2003. "The First 'Award to Active Cities Contest' for the Region of the Americas." *Revista Panamericana de Salud Pública* 14(4): 277–80.

NIHCM (National Institute for Health Care Management). 2003. "Childhood Obesity: Advancing Effective Prevention and Treatment: An Overview for Health Professionals." Washington DC: Prepared for the National Institute for Health Care Management Foundation Forum.

Nugent, Rachel. 2004. "Food and Agriculture Policy: Issues Related to Prevention of Noncommunicable Diseases." *Food and Nutrition Bulletin* 25(2): 200–207.

Orbach, Eliezer, and Gedion Nkojo. 1999. "Assessing the Treatment of Capacity in Africa Region Projects." Washington DC: World Bank.

Osrin, David, Anjana Vaidya, Yagya Shrestha, Ram Bahadur Baniya, Dharma Sharna Manandhar, Ramesh K. Adhikari, and others. 2005. "Effects of Antenatal Multiple Micronutrient Supplementation on Birthweight and Gestational Duration in Nepal: Double-Blind, Randomized Controlled Trial." *Lancet* 365: 955–62.

Panneth, N., and Susser M. 1995. "Early origin of coronary heart disease (the 'Barker hypothesis')." BMJ 310: 411–412.

Pelletier, David L., Edward Frongillo, and Jean-Pierre Habicht. 1994. "Epidemiologic Evidence for a Potentiating Effect of Malnutrition on Child Mortality." *American Journal of Public Health* 83(8): 1130–33.

Pelletier, David L., M. Shekar, and L. Du. Forthcoming. "Bangladesh Integrated Nutrition Project: Effectiveness and Lessons." South Asia Region Human Development, and Human Development Network, World Bank.

Pelletier, David L., Kassahun Deneke, Yemane Kidane, Beyenne Haile, and Fikre Negussie. 1995. "The Food-First Bias and Nutrition Policy: Lessons from Ethiopia." *Food Policy* 20(4): 279–98.

Pollitt, Ernesto. 1990. *Malnutrition and Infection in the Classroom.* Paris: UNESCO.

Popkin, Barry M., Susan Horton, and Soowon Kim. 2001. "The Nutritional Transition and Diet-Related Chronic Diseases in Asia: Implications for Prevention." Washington, DC: International Food Policy Research Institute FCND Discussion Paper 105.

Prentice, Andrew M. 2003. "Intrauterine Factors, Adiposity, and Hyperinsulinaemia." *British Medical Journal* 327:880–81.

Puska, Pekka, Pirjo Pietinen, and Ulla Uusitalo. 2002. "Influencing Public
    Nutrition for Noncommunicable Disease Prevention: From Community
    Intervention to National Programme—Experiences from Finland."
    Public Health Nutrition 5(1A): 245–51.
Puska, Pekka, E. Vartiainen, J. Tuomilehto, V. Salomaa, and A. Nissinen.
    1998. "Changes in Premature Deaths in Finland: Successful Long-Term
    Prevention of Cardiovascular Diseases." *Bulletin of the World Health
    Organization* 76(4): 419–25.
Quisumbing, Agnes R. 2003. "Food Aid and Child Nutrition in Rural
    Ethiopia." Washington, DC: International Food Policy Research Institute
    FCND Discussion Paper 158.
Radhakrishna, R., and K. Subbarao. 1997. *India's Public Distribution System:
    A National and International Perspective.* Washington, DC: World Bank.
Ranatunga, P. 2000. *A Government/Non-Government Collaboration in Poverty
    Alleviation—with a Nutrition Entry.* Self-published.
Ravelli, Anita C.J., Jan H.P. van der Meulen, Clive Osmond, David J.P.
    Barker, and Otto P. Bleker. 1999. "Obesity at the Age of 50 Years in Men
    and Women Exposed to Famine Prenatally." *American Journal of Clinical
    Nutrition* 70: 811–16.
Ravelli, Anita C.J., Jan H.P. van der Meulen, R.P.J. Michels, Clive Osmond,
    David J.P. Barker, C.N. Hales, and Otto P. Bleker. 1998. "Glucose
    Tolerance in Adults after Prenatal Exposure to the Dutch Famine."
    Lancet 351: 173–77.
Ravelli, G.P., Z.A. Steing, M.W. Susser. 1976. "Obesity in young men after
    famine exposure in utero and early infancy." *N Engl J Med* 295:349–53.
Rawlings, Laura B. 2004. "A New Approach to Social Assistance: Latin
    America's Experience with Conditional Cash Transfer Programs."
    Washington, DC: World Bank Social Protection Discussion Paper 416.
Reinikka, Ritva, and Jakob Svensson. 2004. "Local Capture: Evidence from
    a Central Government Transfer Program in Uganda." *Quarterly Journal
    of Economics* 119(2):679–705.
Republic of Uganda–Ministry of Health. 2004. *Nutritional Care and Support
    for People Living with HIV/AIDS in Uganda Guidelines for Service Providers.*
    Kampala: STD/AIDS Control Program.
Richards, Marcus, Rebecca Hardy, Diana Kuh, and Michael E.J. Wadsworth.
    2001. "Birth Weight and Cognitive Function in the British 1946 Birth
    Cohort: Longitudinal Population Based Study." *British Medical Journal*
    322: 199–203.
———. 2002. "Birthweight, Postnatal Growth, and Cognitive Function in
    a National UK Birth Cohort." *International Journal of Epidemiology* 31:
    342–48.
Rivera, Juan A., Daniela Sotres-Alvarez, Jean-Pierre Habicht, Teresa Shamah,
    and Salvador Villalpando. 2004. "Impact of the Mexican Program for

Education, Health, and Nutrition (PROGRESA) on Rates of Growth and Anemia in Infants and Young Children: A Randomized Effectiveness Study." *Journal of the American Medical Association* 29121: 2563–2641.

Rogers, Beatrice Lorge, and Jennifer Coates. 2002. "Food-Based Safety Nets and Related Programs." Washington, DC: World Bank Social Protection Discussion Paper 0223.

Rokx, Claudia. 2000. "Who Should Implement Nutrition Interventions?" Washington, DC: World Bank HNP Discussion Paper.

Roseboom, T.J., J.H. van der Meulen, C. Osmond, D.J. Barker, and others. 2000. "Coronary Heart Disease after Prenatal Exposure to the Dutch Famine, 1944–45." *Heart* 84(6):595–98.

Ross, Jay S., and Miriam H. Labbok. 2004. "Modeling the Effects of Different Infant Feeding Strategies on Infant Survival and Mother-to-Child Transmission of HIV." *American Journal of Public Health* 94(7): 1174–80.

Sanghvi, Tina, Serigne Diene, John Murray, Rae Galloway, and Ciro Franco. 2003 (revised). "Program Review of Essential Nutrition Actions: Checklist for District Health Services." Arlington, VA: Published for the U.S. Agency for International Development by the Basic Support for Institutionalizing Child Survival (BASICS II) Project.

Sari, Mayang, Martin W. Bloem, Saskia de Pee, Werner J. Schultink, and Soemilah Sastroamidjojo. 2001. "Effect of Iron Fortified Candies on the Iron Status of Children Aged 4–6 Years in East Jakarta, Indonesia." *American Journal of Clinical Nutrition* 73: 1034–39.

SCN (United Nations Standing Committee on Nutrition). 2004. *Fifth Report on the World Nutrition Situation: Nutrition for Improved Development Outcomes.* Geneva: SCN.

Serlemitsos, John A., and Harmony Fusco. 2001. "Vitamin A Fortification of Sugar in Zambia, 1998–2001." Washington, DC: The Most Project. http://www.mostproject.org.

Shekar, Meera, and Y-K. Lee. 2005. "Mainstreaming Nutrition in the Context of the World Bank's Poverty Reduction Strategies. What Does It Take?" Washington, DC: World Bank.

Shekar, Meera, Mercedes de Onis, Monika Blössner, and Glaine Borghi. 2004. "Will Asia Meet the Nutrition Millennium Development Goal? And If It Does, Will It Be Enough?" Department of Nutrition for Health and Development, World Health Organization. Unpublished memo.

Shrimpton, Roger, Cesar G. Victora, Mercedes de Onis, Rosângela Costa Lima, Monika Blössner, and Graeme Clugston. 2001. "The Worldwide Timing of Growth Faltering: Implications for Nutritional Interventions." *Pediatrics* 107: e75.

Smith, Lisa C., and Lawrence Haddad. 2000. "Overcoming Child Malnutrition in Developing Countries: Past Achievements and Future

234

REPOSITIONING NUTRITION

Choices." Washington, DC: International Food Policy Research Institute, Food, Agriculture, and the Environment Discussion Paper 30.

Smith, Lisa C., Harold Alderman, and Dede Aduayom. 2005. "Food Insecurity in Sub-Saharan Africa: New Estimates from Household Expenditure Surveys." Draft. Washington, DC: International Food Policy Research Institute.

Smith, Lisa C., Usha Ramakrishnan, Aida Ndiaye, Lawrence Haddad, and Reynaldo Martorell. 2003. "The Importance of Women's Status for Child Nutrition in Developing Countries." Washington, DC: International Food Policy Research Institute Research Report 131.

Sothern, Melinda S., J.N. Udall Jr., R. Suskind, A. Vargas, and U. Blecker. 2000. "Weight Loss and Growth Velocity in Obese Children after Very Low Calorie Diet, Exercise, and Behavior Modification." Acta Paediatrica 89(9): 1036–43.

Sothern, Melinda, H. Schumacher, T. von Almen, L. Carlisle, and J.N. Udall Jr. 2002. "Committed to Kids: An Integrated, Four Level Team Approach to Weight Management in Adolescents." Journal of the American Dietetic Association 102(3): S81–S85.

Strauss, John, and Duncan Thomas. 1998. "Health, Nutrition, and Economic Development." Journal of Economic Literature 36(2): 766–817.

te Velde, Saskia J., Jos W.R. Twisk, Willem Van Mechelen, and Han C.G. Kemper. 2003. "Birth Weight, Adult Body Composition, and Subcutaneous Fat Distribution." Obesity Research 11(2): 202–088.

Tennyson, Ros. 2003. The Partnering Toolbook. London and Geneva: The International Business Leaders Forum (IBLF) and the Global Alliance for Improved Nutrition (GAIN).

Timmer, C. Peter, Walter P. Falcon, and Scott R. Pearson. 1983. Food Policy Analysis. Baltimore, MD: Johns Hopkins University Press.

Toh, C.M., S.K. Chew, and C.C. Tan. 2002. "Prevention and Control of Non-communicable Diseases in Singapore: A Review of National Health Promotion Programmes." Singapore Medical Journal 43(7): 333–39.

Tontsirin, Kraisid, and Stuart Gillespie. 1999. "Linking Community-Based Programs and Service Delivery for Improving Maternal and Child Nutrition." Asian Development Review 17(1, 2): 33–64.

Tontsirin, Kraisid, and Pattanee Winichagoon. 1999. "Community-Based Programmes: Success Factors for Public Nutrition derived from Experience of Thailand." Food and Nutrition Bulletin 20(3): 315–322.

Troutt, David Dante. 1993. The Thin Red Line: How the Poor Still Pay More. San Francisco, CA: West Coast Regional Office, Consumers Union of the United States, Inc.

Tuck, Laura, and Kathy Lindert. 1996. "From Universal Food Subsidies to a Self-Targeted Program: A Case Study in Tunisian Reform." Washington, DC: World Bank Discussion Paper 351.

UNICEF (United Nations Children's Fund). 1990. *Strategy for Improved Nutrition of Children and Women in Developing Countries. A UNICEF Policy Review.* New York: UNICEF.

UNICEF and MI (Micronutrient Initiative). 2004a. *Vitamin and Mineral Deficiency: A Global Damage Assessment Report.* Available at http://www.unicef.org/media/files/davos_micronutrient.pdf.

UNICEF and MI. 2004b. *Vitamin and Mineral Deficiency: A Global Progress Report.* Available at http://www.micronutrient.org/reports/reports/Full_e.pdf.

UNICEF and WHO (World Health Organization). 2004. *Low Birth Weight: Country, Regional, and Global Estimates.* New York: UNICEF.

Van Roekel, Karen, Beth Plowman, Marcia Griffiths, Victorio Vivas de Alvarado, J. Matute, and M. Calderon. 2002. *BASICS II Midterm Evaluation of the AIN Program in Honduras, 2000.* Published for the United States Agency for International Development by the Basic Support for Institutionalizing Child Survival Project (BASICS II).

Von Braun, Joachim. 1995. "Agricultural Commercialization: Impacts on Income and Nutrition and Implications for Policy." *Food Policy* 20(3): 187–202.

Vor der Bruegge, Ellen, Joan E. Dickey, and Christopher Dunford. 1997 (updated 1999). *Cost of Education in the Freedom from Hunger Version of Credit with Education.* Davis, CA: Freedom from Hunger Research Paper 6.

Wagstaff, Adam, and Naoko Watanabe. 2001. *Socioeconomic Inequalities in Child Malnutrition in the Developing World.* Washington, DC: World Bank.

World Bank. 1989. Mozambique—Food Security Study. Washington, DC: World Bank.

———. 1994a. *Impact Evaluation Report. India: Tamil Nadu Integrated Nutrition Project.* Washington, DC: World Bank, Operations Evaluation Department.

———. 1994b. *Enriching Lives: Overcoming Vitamin and Mineral Malnutrition in Developing Countries.* Washington, DC: World Bank Development in Practice Series.

———. 1998. *Implementation Completion Report. Sri Lanka: Poverty Alleviation Project.* Washington, DC: World Bank.

———. 1999a. *Consumer Food Subsidy Programs in the MENA Region.* Washington, DC: World Bank Report No. 19561.

———. 1999b. *Implementation Completion Report. Republic of Madagascar: Food Security and Nutrition Project.* Washington, DC: World Bank.

———1999c. "Consumer Food Subsidy Programs in the MENA Region." Report No. 19561-MNA. Washington, DC: World Bank.

————. 2000. *Voices of the Poor: Can Anyone Hear Us?* Washington, DC: World Bank.

————. 2001a. *Implementation Completion Report. People's Republic of China: Iodine Deficiency Disorders Control Project.* Washington, DC: World Bank.

————. 2001b. *Implementation Completion Report. Republic of Senegal: Community Nutrition Project.* Washington, DC: World Bank.

————. 2001c. *India: Improving Household Food and Nutrition Security: Achievements and Challenges Ahead.* Report 20300-IN. Washington, DC: World Bank.

————. 2002a. *Poverty and Nutrition in Bolivia.* Washington, DC: World Bank.

————. 2002b. *Implementation Completion Report. People's Republic of Bangladesh: Integrated Nutrition Project.* Washington, DC: World Bank.

————. 2002c. *School Health at a Glance.* Washington, DC: World Bank HNP at a Glance Series.

————. 2004. *Implementation Completion Report. Republic of Indonesia: Intensified Iodine Deficiency Control Project.* Washington, DC: World Bank.

————. 2005a. *World Development Indicators.* Washington, DC: World Bank.

————. 2005b. *Global Monitoring Report 2005.* Washington, DC: World Bank.

————. 2005c. *Maintaining Momentum toward the MDGs" An Impact Evaluation of Interventions to Improve Maternal and Child Health and Nutrition Outcomes in Bangladesh.* Operations Evaluation Department (OED). Washington, DC: World Bank.

WHO (World Health Organization). 1995. *Physical Status: The Use and Interpretation of Anthropometry. Report of a WHO Expert Committee.* Geneva: WHO Technical Report Series 845.

————. 2000a. *Obesity: Preventing and Managing the Global Epidemic.* Geneva: WHO Obesity Technical Report Series 894.

————. 2000b. *The Management of Nutrition in Major Emergencies.* Geneva: WHO.

————. 2001. *Diet, Physical Activity, and Health.* EB109/14. Geneva: WHO.

————. 2002. *World Health Report 2002: Reducing Risks, Promoting Healthy Life.* Geneva: WHO.

————. 2004. *Global Strategy on Diet, Physical Activity, and Health.* Fifty-seventh World Health Assembly. WHA57.17. Geneva: WHO. Available at http://www.who.int/gb/ebwha/pdf_files/WHA57/A57_R17-en.pdf.

————. 2005a. *Global Strategy on Diet, Physical Activity and Health.* Available at http://www.who.int/dietphysicalactivity/en.

————. 2005b. Obesity and Overweight. Available at http://www.who.int/dietphysicalactivity/publications/facts/obesity/en/.

————. 2005c. Nutrition and HIV/AIDS: Report by the Secretariat. EB115/12. Available at http://www.who.int/gb/ebwha/pdf_files/EB116/B116_12-en.pdf.

Yamano, Takashi, Harold Alderman, and Luc Christiaensen. 2005. "Child Growth, Shocks, and Food Aid in Rural Ethiopia." *American Journal of Agricultural Economics* 87(2): 273–88.

Zatonski, Witold A., Anthony J. McMichael, and John W. Powles. 1998. "Ecological Study of Reasons for Sharp Decline in Mortality from Ischaemic Heart Disease in Poland Since 1991." *British Medical Journal* 316: 1047–51.

Zeitlin, Marian F., Hossein Ghassemi, and Mohamed Mansour. 1990. Positive Deviance in Child Nutrition. Tokyo: United Nations University.

Zhao, Mingfang, Xiao Ou Shu, Fan Jin, Gong Yang, Hong-Lan Li, Da-Ke Liu, and Wanqing Wen. 2002. "Birthweight, Childhood Growth, and Hypertension in Adulthood." *International Journal of Epidemiology* 31: 1043–51.

Zilberman, David. 2005. "Bringing Health into Agricultural Policy." Presentation abstract for the International Health Economics Association World Congress. Barcelona, Spain. July 10–13.

Zlotkin, Stanley H., Claudia Schauer, Anna Christofides, Waseem Sharieff, Mélody C. Tondeur, and S.M. Ziauddin Hyder. 2005. "Micronutrient Sprinkles to Control Childhood Anaemia." *PLoS Medicine* 2(1): e1.

Index